Air Fryer Cookbook for Two [4 Books in 1]

Hundreds of Healthy Air Fryer Recipes to Burn Fat, Feel Good and Raise Body's Energy Together

By

Chef Mirco Miccio

Table of Contents

Air Fryer Cookbook for Summer

Bariatric Air Fryer Cookbook

The Complete Air Fryer Cookbook with Pictures

20. Air Fried Roasted Salsa 264

21. Air Fried Flour Tortilla Bowls 265

22. Air Fried Cheese and Mini Bean Tacos 266

23. Air Fried Lemon Pepper Shrimp 267

24. Air Fried Shrimp a la Bang Bang 268

25. Air Fried Spicy Bay Scallops 269

26. Air Fried Breakfast Fritatta...270

27. Air Fried Roasted Okra 271

28. Air Fried Rib-Eye Steak 272

29. Air Fried Potato Chips 273

30. Air Fried Tofu 274

31. Air Fried Acorn Squash Slices 275

32. Air Fried Red Potatoes 276

33. Air Fried Butter Cake 277

34. Air Fried Jelly and Peanut Butter S'mores 278

35. Air Fried Sun-Dried Tomatoes 279

36. Air Fried Sweet Potatoes Tots 280

37. Air Fried Banana Bread 281

38. Air Fried Avocado Fries 282

39. "Strawberry Pop Tarts" in an Air Fryer 283

40. Lighten up Empanadas in an Air Fryer 284

41. Air Fried Calzones..286

42. Air Fried Mexican Style Corns 287

43. Air Fryer Crunchy & Crispy Chocolate Bites 288

44. Doritos-Crumbled Chicken tenders in an Air fryer 289

46. Air Fryer Lemonade Scones 291

47. Air Fryer Baked Potatoes...292

48. Air Fryer Mozzarella Chips...293

49. Air Fryer Fetta Nuggets 294

50. Air Fryer Japanese Chicken Tender 295

51. Whole-Wheat Pizzas in an Air Fryer..296

52. Air Fryer Crispy Veggie Quesadillas..297

53. Air Fried Curry Chickpeas 298

Air Fryer Cookbook for Summer

Plenty of Succulent Oil Free Recipes to Eat with Style, Save Your Money and Enjoy the Summertime

By

Chef Mirco Miccio

Table of Contents

Introduction

Most of the people these days like fried food but are afraid of the excessive use of oil. They do not want to disturb their health but they love dishes like fried chips, chicken wings, fried potatoes, grilled seafood and sandwiches, baked muffins, cakes, etc.

Before Air Fryer

They spent money on a separate oven and a grill and a fryer. But guess what you do not need to spend money in all those. Your three in one fryer is here. Many fryers are uncovered and the popping and exploding of oil results in many burns on your skin and is a mess to clean up after you finish. These things may make you not to cook again but not anymore.

Imagine getting your favorite fried food with fewer fats and more healthy nutrients. Your life will be so much better after getting an Air Fryer.

What is an air fryer?

I'm sure you have come across television ads and infomercials showcasing people using an air fryer, and wondered what it is all about. Well, as the name suggests, an air fryer is a device that makes use of air to cook foods.

It basically works by circulating hot air around the food thereby cooking it effectively. It makes use of a fan that produces and circulates the air around the food.

How Does The Air Fryer Work?

The air fryer is a convenient little device that can be used to cook food at a faster pace. Here is looking at the basic functioning of the air fryer

Must Have Air Fryer Accessories
The air fryer looks like a rice cooker, and comes with 3 distinct parts. The first part is the machine itself, which will work by generating hot air that cooks the food within the fryer. The second is the attachment that will carry the food item. The frying basket is the most commonly used attachment. You will also avail a basic pan and a baking tin. The third component is the container. The container holds on to all unwanted food residue such as oil and spices.

The front of the machine carries the temperature and timer that can be adjusted according to the food to be cooked. The insides of the main machine are made up of 5 distinct parts. The back of the machine comes with the water tank. The top of the machine has 4 parts starting with a heating element at the bottom followed by the heating fan, followed by the cooling fan and then the engine.

The main body of the machine might look a little different depending on the brand but most of them pretty much look the same from the inside.

Chapter 1: Benefits Of Air Frying

There are many reasons to use a fryer.

1. Cook healthier
So, how can frying be healthy? Easy! These units can be used without oil or with a small oil jet.

You can cook fries, onion rings, wings and more while getting really crisp results without extra oil. Compared to using my oven, the fries in the fryer were crisper but not dried out, and their use to cook breaded zucchini was even more impressive!

2. Versatility
Depending on the size of your fryer you can buy many accessories. Cake and pizza pans, kebab skewers and steamer are just some of the accessories I've seen.

3. Space saver
If you have a small kitchen or live in a dorm or shared apartment, you can appreciate this benefit. Most of these units are about the size of a coffee machine. They do not take up too much space on the counter and are generally easy to store or move.

Top Reasons Everyone Should Own An Air Fryer

1. Ease of use
Most fryers are very easy to use. Just choose the temperature and cooking time, add food and shake several times during cooking.

With the baskets you can shake your food easily and quickly and the device does not lose much heat when opened. So do not hesitate to check out if you want! Unlike an oven, you will not slow things down when you do it.

2. Easy cleaning
Part of the cooking that most of us do not appreciate is the cleaning. With an air fryer, you only have one basket and one pan to clean, and you can also use dishwasher. With non-stick coated parts, food does not normally stick to the pan. It only takes a few minutes to wash after use. It inspires me to cook more often at home, because I'm not afraid to clean!

3. Energy efficiency
These fryers are more efficient than using an oven. I used mine during a heat wave and I love that my kitchen is not hot when I use it. If you're trying to keep your home cool in the summer or worry about your electricity bills, you'll be impressed with the efficiency of these devices.

How To Use An Air Fryer

•Firstly, you are able to set the temperature based on the thing you need and allow it to preheat for just a few minutes before you decide to place the food in.

•Then open it up and put the meals within the air fryer. Close it and allow the food prepare based on the timing you've set. It will not take enough time regardless of what you're cooking.

•You may use a little bit of cooking spray or splash some oil around the food before putting it in. This can help to prevent the meals from getting stuck towards the pan. The oil likewise helps to create food a bit crispier and provides the taste of standard fried food.

•Halfway with the set time or perhaps in between times, provide the air fryer just a little shake so the air inside circulates easily and your meals are completely cooked.

•Other than frying, you can test other cooking methods while using additional parts the air flyers usually include. You should use the grill or baking tray in compliance using the instructions that include the environment fryer.

•Another factor to bear in mind is you shouldn't overcrowd the fryer by putting an excessive amount of food inside it. Put small batches of food within the air fryer to ensure that there's enough room for this all to maneuver and prepare evenly. Overcrowding won't let it move and a few parts is going to be left uncooked. The cooking can also be elevated if you devote an excessive amount of at the same time.

•In the situation of marinated food, allow it to be as dry as you possibly can before placing it within the air fryer. Wet food may cause splattering in addition to an excessive amount of smoke being released in the fryer.

•The separator that will get the environment fryer can be put among layers of food in order to prepare various things concurrently. Just make certain the temperature needed is identical for those products or they will not be cooked evenly.

•Pre-packaged meals may also be made while using air fryer. Lower the suggested oven temperature and hang the environment fryer after your meals are placed within it. Additionally, it cuts down on the normal cooking considerably.

•For baking food, you should use the baking pan provided or purchase one individually. You do not need a stove to bake some muffins any longer and also you have them cooked even faster than in the past.

•Roasting meals are also simpler than using conventional methods. It doesn't take considerable time but you just get individuals healthy and attractive roasted veggies or meats that you simply love. For grilling food, put the grill layer inside as well as your food on the top from it. You don't need to help keep flipping the meals over as with a conventional grill.

This will make things much easier. Give it a shake following a couple of moments for much better air flow. As possible clearly see in the information above, significantly less efforts are needed while the food is cooking. Make use of the simple mechanism and prepare a number of different meals every single day. They get cooked in almost no time and taste great.

Chapter 2: Air Fryer Tips And Tricks

The air fryer makes use of the same technology and causes the amino acids and sugar in the foods to react and develop a brown color.

The mechanism makes the food crispy on the outside, thereby giving it the feeling of a baked or fried food item.

The air fryer is capable of raising the air temperature to up to 200 degree Celsius, which means it permeates through the food to cook it thoroughly.

Here are the different things you can do with an air fryer.

Frying

Now you don't have to worry about deep-frying foods, as it is quite easy to use an air fryer to get the desired results. In fact, you don't need any oil at all to fry the foods, as the fryer makes use of hot air to crisp up foods. All you have to do is add in a little oil to the ingredient mix, which the air fryer will use to both cook and crisp the food. You can, however, brush a little oil on top to make it a little crunchier if you like.

Grilling

It is extremely easy to grill in an air fryer and you only have to expend a little effort towards it. You don't have to worry about constantly flipping the food, as all you have to do is add the food and wait. Once you reach the half way mark, you can give the fryer a gentle shake in order to readjust the food within it. You will have to use the grill attachment, as that will make it easy for you to move the food by using the handle attached to it. The shaking also helps with absorbing or draining the excess oil, thereby making the food healthier.

Baking

Baking is made extremely easy with the air fryer. You don't have to worry about not having a conventional oven, as the air fryer will work well for all your baking needs. It works on pretty much the same rules as an oven and you have to preheat it before baking.

Roasting

This is the most used function of the air fryer. It will be extremely easy for you to roast your foods as the air fryer works very fast. All you have to do is prepare the vegetables or meats by cutting them into small pieces and then add them to the roasting attachment. You don't have to worry about turning or moving them around, as the air fryer will do all the work for you. The air fryer takes 20% lesser time to roast your vegetables and meats, which makes it great for bachelors, and those in a hurry to cook their food.

Air Fryer Cleaning & Maintenance

It is important for you to clean the air fryer from time to time to ensure that it serves you for as long as possible. Here are the simple steps that you can adopt to clean and maintain the air fryer.

- To clean the cooking basket start by filling a large enough tub with hot water and detergent to generate thick foam.

- Place the attachment within it and allow it to soak for a while before using a brush to clean it thoroughly.

- But be careful so as to not scrub it using harsh brushes as they can leave behind scratches.

- The outside of an air fryer will not get as greasy as a conventional fryer. All you have to do is wipe it with a damp cloth and your fryer will be as good as new.

- You can dip the cloth in hot water if you wish to loosen a stain.

- If there is a tough stain then you can use a toothbrush dipped in salt to scrub over the stain.

- But make sure you don't use a steel mesh or a hard bristled toothbrush as they can leave behind scratches on the body of the machine.

- You must also clean the basket at the bottom that catches the residue. You must empty it as soon as you finish the cooking and pop it into the dishwasher to clean it or follow the same procedure as you would to clean the attachment.

Money saving tips

As Air fryer requires less oil, you wouldn't need to buy huge packets of oils in your monthly groceries. This would lessen your grocery bills. You do not need to buy griller, fryer, and an oven separately. This is your all in one rounder. Remember the dress you wanted to take? But unfortunately, you could not buy it. Not anymore. Not only your grocery bills will decrease, you will witness an immense change in your gas bills. As air fryer makes the oil hot in one-third time of other fryers and your stove will require less gas. The lesser you will utilize gas the lesser your bill will be. This will save the money that you were going to spend on a griller and oven.

A cosmic amount will be saved and you do not need to see your favorite dress cashed by someone else. Not only dresses, you can get whatever you want. Air fryer is an efficient and smart choice for everyone. Air fryer would give you an ease and this would save your time and money even health too. Who would not want to get such an opportunity?

Chapter 3: Air Fryer Breakfast Recipes

No-Bun Breakfast Bacon Burger

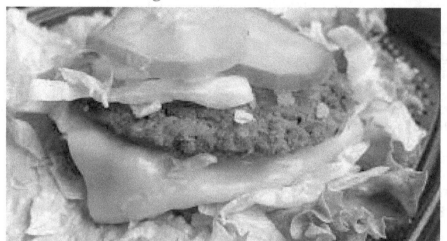

Cook Time: 8 minutes

Servings: 2

Ingredients:

8-ounces ground beef

2-ounces lettuce leaves

½ teaspoon minced garlic

1 teaspoon olive oil

½ teaspoon sea salt

1 teaspoon ground black pepper

1 teaspoon butter

4-ounces bacon, cooked

1 egg

½ yellow onion, diced

½ cucumber, slice finely

½ tomato, slice finely

Directions:

Begin by whisking the egg in a bowl, then add the ground beef and combine well. Add cooked, chopped bacon to the ground beef mixture. Add butter, ground black pepper, minced garlic, and salt. Mix and make burgers. Preheat your air fryer to 370°Fahrenheit.

Spray the air fryer basket with olive oil and place the burgers inside of it. Cook the burgers for 8-minutes on each side. Meanwhile, slice the cucumber, onion, and tomato finely. Place the tomato, onion, and cucumber onto the lettuce leaves. When the burgers are cooked, allow them to chill at room temperature, and place them over the vegetables and serve.

Nutritional Values per serving: Calories: 618, Total Fat: 37.8g, Carbs: 8.6g, Protein: 59.4g

Scrambled Pancake Hash

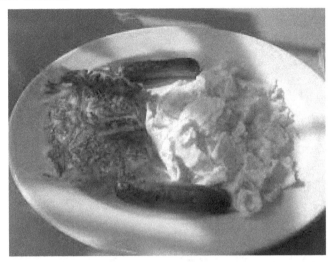

Cook Time: 9 minutes

Servings: 7

Ingredients:

1 egg

¼ cup heavy cream

5 tablespoons butter

1 cup coconut flour

1 teaspoon ground ginger

1 teaspoon salt

1 tablespoon apple cider vinegar

1 teaspoon baking soda

Directions:

Combine the salt, baking soda, ground ginger and flour in a mixing bowl. In a separate bowl crack, the egg into it. Add butter and heavy cream. Mix well using a hand mixer.

Combine the liquid and dry mixtures and stir until smooth. Preheat your air fryer to 400°Fahrenheit. Pour the pancake mixture into the air fryer basket tray. Cook the pancake hash for 4-minutes. After this, scramble the pancake hash well and continue to cook for another 5-minutes more. When dish is cooked, transfer it to serving plates, and serve hot!

Nutritional Values per serving: Calories: 178, Total Fat: 13.3g, Carbs: 10.7g, Protein: 4.4g

Morning Time Sausages

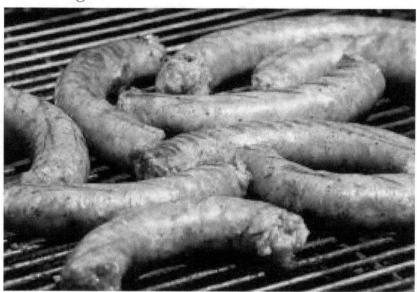

Cook Time: 12 minutes

Servings: 6

Ingredients:

7-ounces ground chicken

7-ounces ground pork

1 teaspoon ground coriander

1 teaspoon basil, dried

½ teaspoon nutmeg

1 teaspoon olive oil

1 teaspoon minced garlic

1 tablespoon coconut flour

1 egg

1 teaspoon soy sauce

1 teaspoon sea salt

½ teaspoon ground black pepper

Directions:

Combine the ground pork, chicken, soy sauce, ground black pepper, garlic, basil, coriander, nutmeg, sea salt, and egg. Add the coconut flour and mix the mixture well to combine. Preheat your air fryer to 360°Fahrenheit. Make medium-sized sausages with the ground meat mixture. Spray the inside of the air fryer basket tray with the olive oil. Place prepared sausages into the air fryer basket and place inside of air fryer. Cook the sausages for 6-minutes. Turn the sausages over and cook for 6-minutes more. When the cook time is completed, let the sausages chill for a little bit. Serve warm.

Nutritional Values per serving: Calories: 156, Total Fat: 7.5g, Carbs: 1.3g, Protein: 20.2g

Breakfast Meatloaf Slices

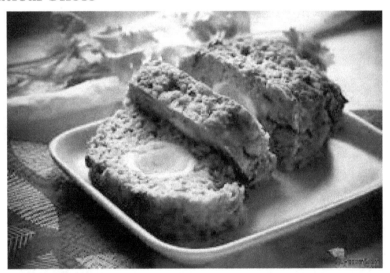

Cook Time: 20 minutes

Servings: 6

Ingredients:

8-ounces ground pork

7-ounces ground beef

1 teaspoon olive oil

1 teaspoon butter

1 tablespoon oregano, dried

1 teaspoon cayenne pepper

1 teaspoon salt

1 tablespoon chives

1 tablespoon almond flour

1 egg

1 onion, diced

Directions:

Beat egg in a bowl. Add the ground beef and ground pork. Add the chives, almond flour, cayenne pepper, salt, dried oregano, and butter. Add diced onion to ground beef mixture. Use hands to shape a meatloaf mixture. Preheat the air fryer to 350°Fahrenheit. Spray the inside of the air fryer basket with olive oil and place the meatloaf inside it. Cook the meatloaf for 20-minutes. When the meatloaf has cooked, allow it to chill for a bit. Slice and serve it.

Nutritional Values per serving: Calories: 176, Total Fat: 6.2g, Carbs: 3.4g, Protein: 22.2g

Egg Butter

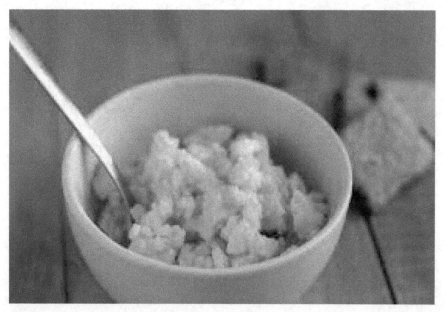

Cook Time: 17 minutes

Servings: 4

Ingredients:

4 eggs

4 tablespoons butter

1 teaspoon salt

Directions:

Cover the air fryer basket with foil and place the eggs there. Transfer the air fryer basket into the air fryer and cook the eggs for 17 minutes at 320°Fahrenheit. When the time is over, remove the eggs from the air fryer basket and put them in cold water to chill them. After this, peel the eggs and chop them up finely. Combine the chopped eggs with butter and add salt. Mix it until you get the spread texture. Serve the egg butter with the keto almond bread.

Nutritional Values per serving: Calories: 164, Total Fat: 8.5g, Carbs: 2.67g, Protein: 3g

Kale Breakfast Fritters

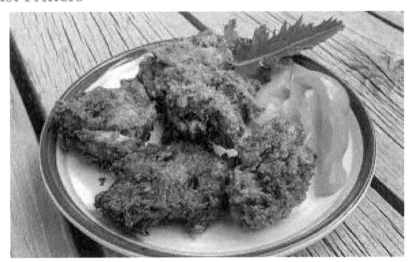

Cook Time: 8 minutes

Servings: 8

Ingredients:

12-ounces kale, chopped

1 teaspoon oil

1 tablespoon cream

1 teaspoon paprika

½ teaspoon sea salt

2 tablespoons almond flour

1 egg

1 tablespoon butter

½ yellow onion, diced

Directions:

Wash and chop the kale. Add the chopped kale to blender and blend it until smooth. Dice up the yellow onion. Beat the egg and whisk it in a mixing bowl. Add the almond flour, paprika, cream and salt into bowl with whisked egg and stir. Add the diced onion and blended kale to mixing bowl and mix until you get fritter dough. Preheat your air fryer to 360°Fahrenheit. Spray the inside of the air fryer basket with olive oil. Make medium-sized fritters with prepared mixture and place them into air fryer basket. Cook the kale fritters 4-minutes on each side. Once they are cooked, allow them to chill then serve.

Nutritional Values per serving:, Calories: 86, Total Fat: 5.6g, Carbs: 6.8g, Protein: 3.6g

Seed Porridge

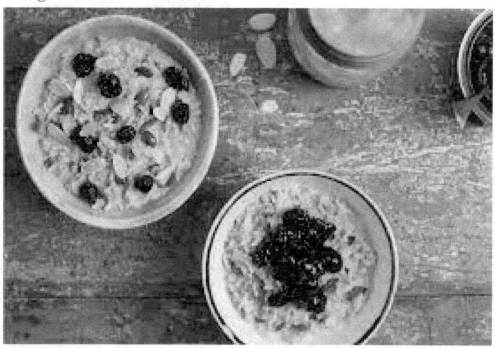

Cook Time: 12 minutes

Servings: 3

Ingredients:

1 tablespoon butter

¼ teaspoon nutmeg

1/3 cup heavy cream

1 egg

¼ teaspoon salt

3 tablespoons sesame seeds

3 tablespoons chia seeds

Directions:

Place the butter in your air fryer basket tray. Add the chia seeds, sesame seeds, heavy cream, nutmeg, and salt. Stir gently. Beat the egg in a cup and whisk it with a fork. Add the whisked egg to air fryer basket tray. Stir the mixture with a wooden spatula. Preheat your air fryer to 375°Fahrenheit. Place the air fryer basket tray into air fryer and cook the porridge for 12-minutes. Stir it about 3 times during the cooking process. Remove the porridge from air fryer basket tray immediately and serve hot!

Nutritional Values per serving: Calories: 275, Total Fat: 22.5g, Carbs: 13.2g, Protein: 7.9g

Keto Bread-Free Breakfast Sandwich

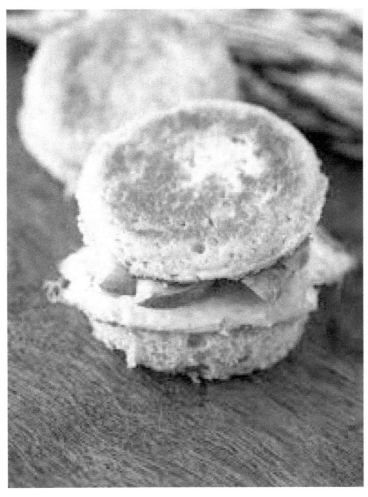

Cook Time: 10 minutes

Servings: 2

Ingredients:

6-ounces ground chicken

2 slices of cheddar cheese

2 lettuce leaves

1 tablespoon dill, dried

½ teaspoon sea salt

1 egg

1 teaspoon cayenne pepper

1 teaspoon tomato puree

Directions:

Combine the ground chicken with the pepper and sea salt. Add the dried dill and stir. Beat the egg into the ground chicken mixture. Make 2 medium-sized burgers from the ground chicken mixture. Preheat your air fryer to 380°Fahrenheit. Spray the air fryer basket tray with olive oil and place the ground chicken burgers inside of it. Cook the chicken burgers for 10-minutes. Flip over burgers and cook for an additional 6-minutes. When the burgers are cooked, transfer them to the lettuce leaves. Sprinkle the top of them with tomato puree and with a slice of cheddar cheese. Serve immediately!

Nutritional Values per serving: Calories: 324, Total Fat: 19.2g, Carbs: 2.3g, Protein: 34.8g

Breakfast Liver Pate

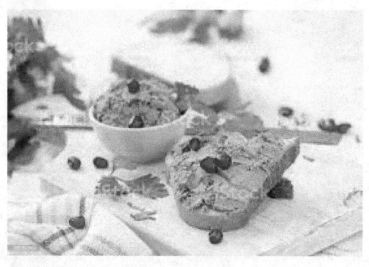

Cook Time: 10 minutes

Servings: 7

Ingredients:

1 lb. chicken liver

1 teaspoon salt

½ teaspoon cilantro, dried

1 yellow onion, diced

1 teaspoon ground black pepper

1 cup water

4 tablespoons butter

Directions:

Chop the chicken liver roughly and place it in the air fryer basket tray. Add water to air fryer basket tray and add diced onion. Preheat your air fryer to 360°Fahrenheit and cook chicken liver for 10-minutes. When it is finished cooking, drain the chicken liver. Transfer the chicken liver to blender, add butter, ground black pepper and dried cilantro and blend. Once you get a pate texture, transfer to liver pate bowl and serve immediately or keep in the fridge for later.

Nutritional Values per serving: Calories: 173, Total Fat: 10.8g, Carbs: 2.2g, Protein: 16.1g

Eggs in Zucchini Nests

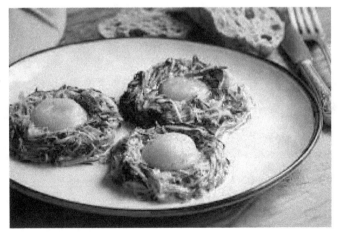

Cook Time: 7 minutes

Servings: 4

Ingredients:

4 teaspoons butter

½ teaspoon paprika

½ teaspoon black pepper

¼ teaspoon sea salt

4-ounces cheddar cheese, shredded

4 eggs

8-ounces zucchini, grated

Directions:

Grate the zucchini and place the butter in ramekins. Add the grated zucchini in ramekins in the shape of nests. Sprinkle the zucchini nests with salt, pepper, and paprika. Beat the eggs and pour over zucchini nests. Top egg mixture with shredded cheddar cheese. Preheat the air fryer basket and cook the dish for 7-minutes. When the zucchini nests are cooked, chill them for 3-minutes and serve them in the ramekins.

Nutritional Values per serving: Calories: 221, Total Fat: 17.7g, Carbs: 2.9g, Protein: 13.4g

Breakfast Chicken Hash

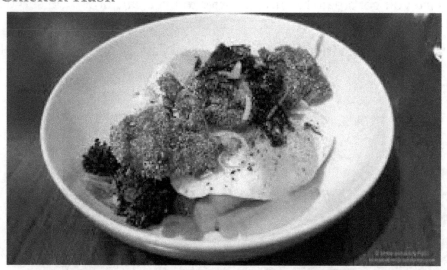

Cook Time: 14 minutes

Servings: 3

Ingredients:

6-ounces of cauliflower, chopped

7-ounce chicken fillet

1 tablespoon water

1 green pepper, chopped

½ yellow onion, diced

1 teaspoon ground black pepper

3 tablespoons butter

1 tablespoon cream

Directions:

Chop the cauliflower and place into the blender and blend it carefully until you get cauliflower rice. Chop the chicken fillet into small pieces. Sprinkle the chicken fillet with ground black pepper and stir. Preheat your air fryer to 380°Fahrenheit. Dice the yellow onion and chop the green pepper. In a large mixing bowl, combine ingredients, then add mixture to fryer basket. Then cook and serve chicken hash warm!

Nutritional Values per serving: Calories: 261, Total Fat: 16.8g, Carbs: 7.1g, Protein: 21g

Flax Meal Porridge

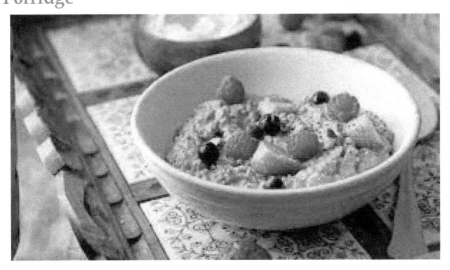

Cook Time: 8 minutes

Servings: 4

Ingredients:

2 tablespoons sesame seeds

½ teaspoon vanilla extract

1 tablespoon butter

1 tablespoon liquid Stevia

3 tablespoons flax meal

1 cup almond milk

4 tablespoons chia seeds

Directions:

Preheat your air fryer to 375°Fahrenheit. Put the sesame seeds, chia seeds, almond milk, flax meal, liquid Stevia and butter into the air fryer basket tray. Add the vanilla extract and cook porridge for 8-minutes. When porridge is cooked stir it carefully then allow it to rest for 5-minutes before serving.

Nutritional Values per serving: Calories: 298, Total Fat: 26.7g, Carbs: 13.3 g, Protein: 6.2g

Breakfast Chicken Strips

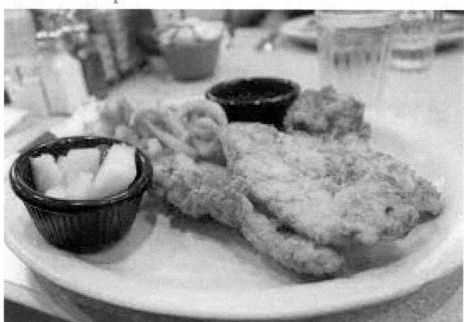

Cook Time: 12 minutes

Servings: 4

Ingredients:

1 teaspoon paprika

1 tablespoon cream

1 lb. chicken fillet

½ teaspoon salt

½ teaspoon black pepper

Directions:

Cut the chicken fillet into strips. Sprinkle the chicken fillets with salt and pepper. Preheat the air fryer to 365°Fahrenheit. Place the butter in the air basket tray and add the chicken strips. Cook the chicken strips for 6-minutes. Turn the chicken strips to the other side and cook them for an additional 5-minutes. After strips are cooked, sprinkle them with cream and paprika, then transfer them to serving plates. Serve warm.

Nutritional Values per serving: Calories: 245, Total Fat: 11.5g, Carbs: 0.6g, Protein: 33g

Breakfast Hash

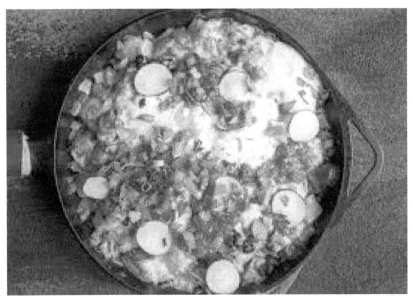

Cook Time: 8 minutes

Servings: 4

Ingredients:

7-ounces bacon, cooked

1 zucchini, cubed into small pieces

4-ounces cheddar cheese, shredded

2 tablespoons butter

1 teaspoon ground thyme

1 teaspoon cilantro

1 teaspoon paprika

1 teaspoon ground black pepper

1 teaspoon salt

Directions:

Chop the zucchini into small cubes and sprinkle with ground black pepper, salt, paprika, cilantro and ground thyme. Preheat your air fryer to 400°Fahrenheit. Add butter to the air fryer basket tray. Melt the butter and add the zucchini cubes. Cook the zucchini cubes for 5-minutes. Meanwhile, shred the cheddar cheese. Add the bacon to the zucchini cubes. Sprinkle the zucchini mixture with shredded cheese and cook for 3-minutes more. When cooking is completed, transfer the breakfast hash into serving bowls.

Nutritional Values per serving: Calories: 445, Total Fat: 36.1g, Carbs: 3.5g, Protein: 26.3g

Keto Air Bread

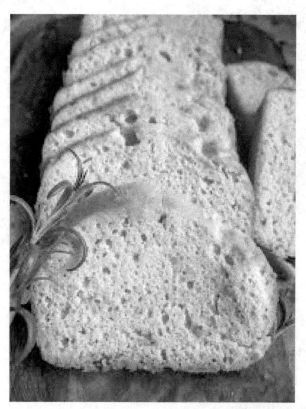

Cook Time: 25 minutes

Servings: 19

Ingredients:

1 cup almond flour

¼ sea salt

1 teaspoon baking powder

¼ cup butter

3 eggs

Directions:

Crack the eggs into a bowl then using a hand blender mix them up. Melt the butter at room temperature. Take the melted butter and add it to the egg mixture. Add the salt, baking powder and almond flour to egg mixture and knead the dough. Cover the prepared dough with a towel for 10-minutes to rest. Meanwhile, preheat your air fryer to 360°Fahrenheit. Place the prepared dough in the air fryer tin and cook the bread for 10-minutes. Then reduce the heat to 350°Fahrenheit and cook the bread for an additional 15-minutes. You can use a toothpick to check to make sure the bread is cooked. Transfer the bread to a wooden board to allow it to chill. Once the bread has chilled, then slice and serve it.

Nutritional Values per serving: Calories: 40, Total Fat: 3.9g, Carbs: 0.5g, Protein: 1.2g

Herbed Breakfast Eggs

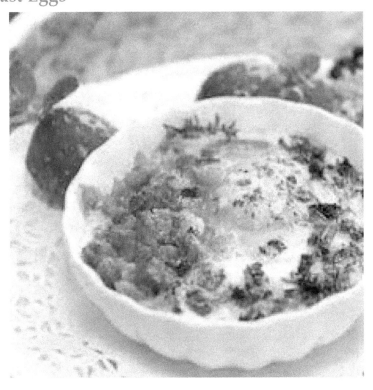

Cook Time: 17 minutes

Servings: 2

Ingredients:

4 eggs

1 teaspoon oregano

1 teaspoon parsley, dried

½ teaspoon sea salt

1 tablespoon chives, chopped

1 tablespoon cream

1 teaspoon paprika

Directions:

Place the eggs in the air fryer basket and cook them for 17-minutes at 320°Fahrenheit. Meanwhile, combine the parsley, oregano, cream, and salt in shallow bowl. Chop the chives and add them to cream mixture. When the eggs are cooked, place them in cold water and allow them to chill. After this, peel the eggs and cut them into halves. Remove the egg yolks and add yolks to cream mixture and mash to blend well with a fork. Then fill the egg whites with the cream-egg yolk mixture. Serve immediately.

Nutritional Values per serving: Calories: 136, Total Fat: 9.3g, Carbs: 2.1g, Protein: 11.4g

Baked Bacon Egg Cups

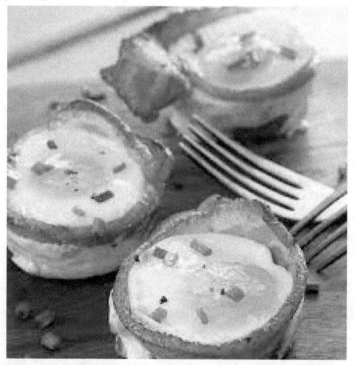

Cooking Time: 12 minutes

Servings: 2

Ingredients:

2 eggs

1 tablespoon chives, fresh, chopped

½ teaspoon paprika

½ teaspoon cayenne pepper

3-ounces cheddar cheese, shredded

½ teaspoon butter

¼ teaspoon salt

4-ounces bacon, cut into tiny pieces

Directions:

Slice bacon into tiny pieces and sprinkle it with cayenne pepper, salt, and paprika. Mix the chopped bacon. Spread butter in bottom of ramekin dishes and beat the eggs there. Add the chives and shredded cheese. Add the chopped bacon over egg mixture in ramekin dishes. Place the ramekins in your air fryer basket. Preheat your air fryer to 360°Fahrenheit. Place the air fryer basket in your air fryer and cook for 12-minutes. When the cook time is completed, remove the ramekins from air fryer and serve warm.

Nutritional Values per serving: Calories: 553, Total Fat: 43.3g, Carbs: 2.3g, Protein: 37.3g

Breakfast Coconut Porridge

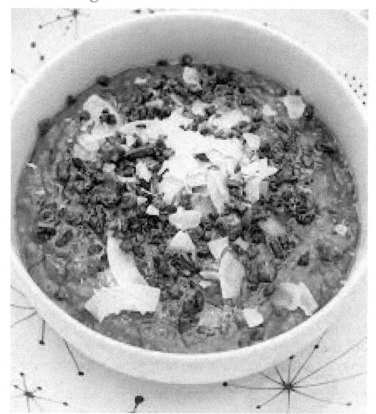

Cook Time: 7 minutes

Servings: 4

Ingredients:
1 cup coconut milk

3 tablespoons blackberries

2 tablespoons walnuts

1 teaspoon butter

1 teaspoon ground cinnamon

5 tablespoons chia seeds

3 tablespoons coconut flakes

¼ teaspoon salt

Directions:

Pour the coconut milk into the air fryer basket tray. Add the coconut, salt, chia seeds, ground cinnamon, and butter. Ground up the walnuts and add them to the air fryer basket tray. Sprinkle the mixture with salt. Mash the blackberries with a fork and add them also to the air fryer basket tray. Cook the porridge at 375°Fahrenheit for 7-minutes. When the cook time is over, remove the air fryer basket from air fryer and allow to sit and rest for 5-minutes. Stir porridge with a wooden spoon and serve warm.

Nutritional Values per serving: Calories: 169, Total Fat: 18.2g, Carbs: 9.3g, Protein: 4.2g

Keto Spinach Quiche

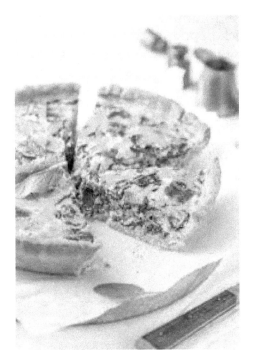

Cook Time: 21 minutes

Servings: 6

Ingredients:

6-ounces cheddar cheese, shredded

1 teaspoon olive oil

3 eggs

1 teaspoon ground black pepper

½ yellow onion, diced

¼ cup cream cheese

1 cup spinach

1 teaspoon sea salt

4 tablespoons water, boiled

½ cup almond flour

Directions:

Combine the almond flour, water, and salt. Mix and knead the dough. Spray the inside of the fryer basket with olive oil. Set your air fryer to 375°Fahrenheit. Roll the dough and place it in your air fryer basket tray in the shape of the crust. Place air fryer basket tray inside of air fryer and cook for 5-minutes. Chop the spinach and combine it with the cream cheese and ground black pepper. Dice the yellow onion and add it to the spinach mixture and stir. Whisk eggs in a bowl. When the quiche crust is cooked — transfer the spinach filling. Sprinkle the filling top with shredded cheese and pour the whisked eggs over the top. Set the air fryer to 350°Fahrenheit. Cook the quiche for 7-minutes. Reduce the heat to 300°Fahrenheit and cook the quiche for an additional 9-minutes. Allow the quiche to chill thoroughly and then cut it into pieces for serving.

Nutritional Values per serving: Calories: 248, Total Fat: 20.2g, Carbs: 4.1g, Protein: 12.8g

Western Omelette

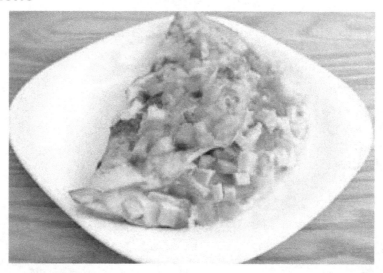

Cook Time: 10 minutes

Servings: 4

Ingredients:

1 green pepper

5 eggs

½ yellow onion, diced

3-ounces Parmesan cheese, shredded

1 teaspoon butter

1 teaspoon oregano, dried

1 teaspoon cilantro, dried

1 teaspoon olive oil

3 tablespoons cream cheese

Directions:

In a bowl, add the eggs and whisk them. Sprinkle the cilantro, oregano, and cream cheese into the eggs. Add the shredded parmesan and mix the egg mixture well. Preheat your air fryer to 360°Fahrenheit. Pour the egg mixture into the air fryer basket tray and place it into the air fryer. Cook the omelet for 10-minutes. Meanwhile, chop the green pepper and dice the onion. Pour olive oil into a skillet and preheat well over medium heat. Add the chopped green pepper and onion to skillet and roast for 8-minutes. Stir veggies often. Remove the omelet from air fryer basket tray and place it on a serving plate. Add the roasted vegetables and serve warm.

Nutritional Values per serving: Calories: 204, Total Fat: 14.9g, Carbs: 4.3g, Protein: 14.8g

Chapter 4: Lunch

Bacon, Lettuce, Tempeh & Tomato Sandwiches

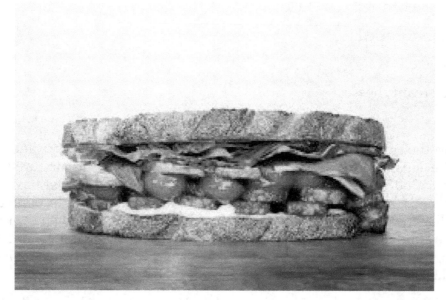

Cook Time: 5 minutes

Servings: 4

Ingredients:

8-ounce package tempeh

1 cup warm vegetable broth

Tomato slices and lettuce, to serve

¼ teaspoon chipotle chili powder

½ teaspoon garlic powder

½ teaspoon onion powder

1 teaspoon Liquid smoke

3 tablespoons soy sauce

Directions:

Begin by opening the packet of tempeh and slice into pieces about ¼ inch thick. Grab a medium bowl and add the remaining ingredients except for lettuce and tomato and stir well. Place the pieces of tempeh onto a baking tray that will fit into your air fryer and pour over the flavor mix. Put the tray in air fryer and cook for 5-minutes at 360°Fahrenheit. Remove from air fryer and place on sliced bread with the tomato and lettuce and any other extra toppings you desire.

Nutritional Values per serving: Carbs: 265, Total Fat: 11.3g, Carbs: 9.2g, Protein: 12.4g

Coconut Chips

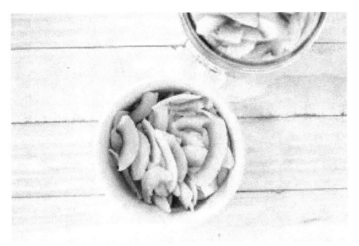

Cook Time: 5 minutes

Servings: 2

Ingredients:

2 cups large pieces of shredded coconut

1/3 teaspoon liquid Stevia

1 tablespoon chili powder

Directions:

Preheat your air fryer to 390°Fahrenheit. Combine the shredded coconut pieces with spices. Cook for 5-minutes in air fryer and enjoy!

Nutritional Values per serving: Calories: 261, Total Fat: 9.2g, Carbs: 7.3g, Protein: 6.2g

Sweet Potato Chips

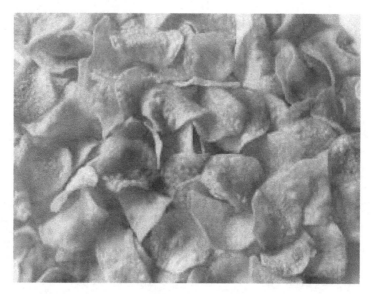

Cook Time: 15 minutes

Servings: 2

Ingredients:

2 large sweet potatoes, thinly sliced with Mandoline

2 tablespoons olive oil

Salt to taste

Directions:

Preheat your air fryer to 350°Fahrenheit. Stir the sweet potato slices, in a large bowl with the oil. Arrange slices in your air fryer and cook them until crispy, for about 15-minutes.

Nutritional Values per serving: Calories: 253, Total Fat: 11.2g, Carbs: 8.4g, Protein: 6.5g

Air Fryer Apple Pork Balls

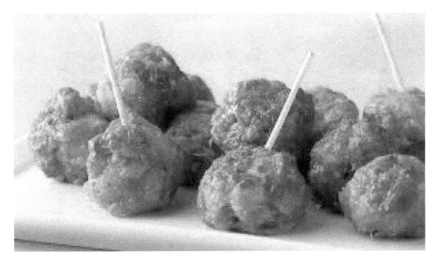

Cook Time: 15 minutes

Servings: 8

Ingredients:

2 teaspoons Dijon mustard

5 basil leaves, chopped

Salt and pepper to taste

2 tablespoons cheddar cheese, grated

4 garlic cloves, minced

1 small apple, chopped

1 large onion, chopped

1 1b. pork, minced

Directions:

Add the minced pork, onion, and apple into mixing bowl and stir. Add mustard, honey, garlic, cheese, basil, pepper, salt and mix well. Make small balls from mixture and place them inside of air fryer basket. Cook at 400°Fahrenheit for 15-minutes.

Nutritional Values per serving: Calories: 267, Total Fat: 12.3g, Carbs: 11.6g, Protein: 16.4g

Air Fryer Pork Loin with Sweet Potatoes

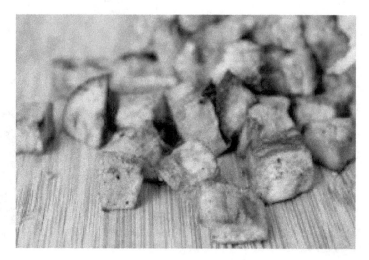

Cook Time: 25 minutes

Servings: 8

Ingredients:

2 lbs. pork loin

2 large Sweet potatoes, diced

1 teaspoon salt

1 teaspoon pepper

½ teaspoon garlic powder

½ teaspoon parsley flakes

Directions:

Add all the ingredients into mixing bowl and mix well.   Add bowl with pork and sweet potato mixture into air fryer basket. Cook in air fryer at 350°Fahrenheit for 25-minutes. Carve up the pork into slices and serve with sweet potatoes.

Nutritional Values per serving: Calories: 286, Total Fat: 12.6g, Carbs: 11.4g, Protein: 16.6g

Onion Pakora

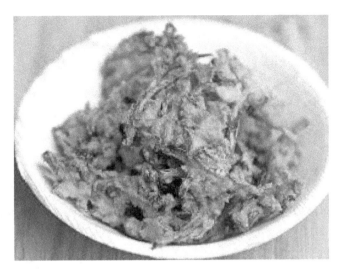

Cook Time: 6 minutes

Servings: 6

Ingredients:

1 cup graham flour

¼ teaspoon turmeric powder

Salt to taste

1/8 teaspoon chili powder

¼ teaspoon carom

1 tablespoon fresh coriander, chopped

2 green chili peppers, finely chopped

4 onions, finely chopped

2 teaspoons vegetable oil

¼ cup rice flour

Directions:

Combine the flours and oil in a mixing bowl. Add water as needed to create a dough-like consistency. Add peppers, onions, coriander, carom, chili powder, and turmeric. Preheat air fryer to 350°Fahrenheit. Roll vegetable mixture into small balls, add to the fryer and cook for about 6-minutes. Serve with hot sauce!

Nutritional Values per serving: Calories: 253, Total Fat: 12.2g, Carbs: 11.4g, Protein: 7.6g

Mushroom, Onion and Feta Frittata

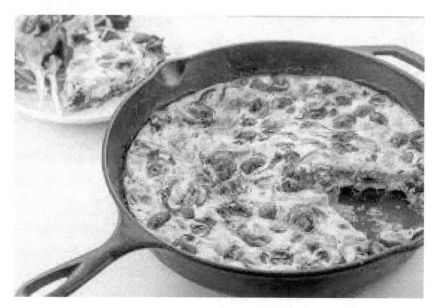

Cook Time: 30 minutes

Servings: 4

Ingredients:

4 cups button mushrooms

1 red onion

2 tablespoons olive oil

6 tablespoons feta cheese, crumbled

Pinch of salt

6 eggs

Cooking spray

Directions:

Peel and slice the red onion into ¼ inch thin slices. Clean the button mushrooms, then cut them into ¼ inch thin slices. Add olive oil to pan and sauté mushrooms over medium heat until tender. Remove from heat and pan so that they can cool. Preheat your air fryer to 330°Fahrenheit. Add cracked eggs into a bowl, and whisk them, adding a pinch of salt. Coat an 8-inch heat resistant baking dish with cooking spray. Add the eggs into the baking dish, then onion and mushroom mixture, and then add feta cheese. Place the baking dish into air fryer for 30-minutes and serve warm.

Nutritional Values per serving: Calories: 246, Total Fat: 12.3g, Carbs: 9.2g, Protein: 10.3g

Curried Cauliflower Florets

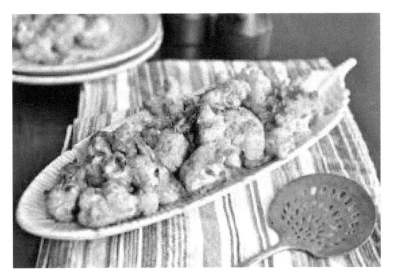

Cook Time: 10 minutes

Servings: 4

Ingredients:

1/4 cup sultanas or golden raisins

¼ teaspoon salt

1 tablespoon curry powder

1 head cauliflower, broken into small florets

¼ cup pine nuts

½ cup olive oil

Directions:

In a cup of boiling water, soak your sultanas to plump. Preheat your air fryer to 350°Fahrenheit. Add oil and pine nuts to air fryer and toast for a minute or so. In a bowl toss the cauliflower and curry powder as well as salt, then add the mix to air fryer mixing well. Cook for 10-minutes. Drain the sultanas, toss with cauliflower, and serve.

Nutritional Values per serving: Calories: 275, Total Fat: 11.3g, Carbs: 8.6g, Protein: 9.5g

Pork Chunks with Sweet & Sour Sauce

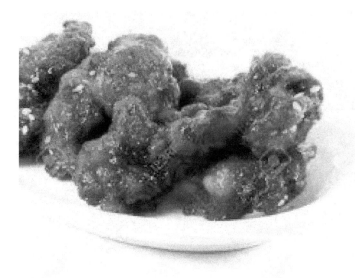

Cook Time: 10 minutes

Servings: 4

Ingredients:

1 cup cornstarch

½ teaspoon spice mix

¼ cup sweet and sour sauce

2 lbs. pork, chunked

3 tablespoons olive oil

2 large eggs, beaten

½ teaspoon sea salt

¼ teaspoon black pepper

Directions:

In a bowl, combine spice mix, cornstarch, pepper, and salt. In another bowl add beaten eggs. Coat pork chunks with cornstarch mixture then dip in eggs and again into cornstarch. Grease air fryer basket with olive oil and preheat to 340°Fahrenheit. Place the coated pork chunks into air fryer basket and cook for 10-minutes. Shake the basket halfway through the cook time. Place the air fried pork chunks on serving dish and drizzle with sweet and sour sauce.

Nutritional Values per serving: Calories: 282, Total Fat: 12.6g, Carbs: 11.5g, Protein: 17.3g

Panko-Crusted Tilapia

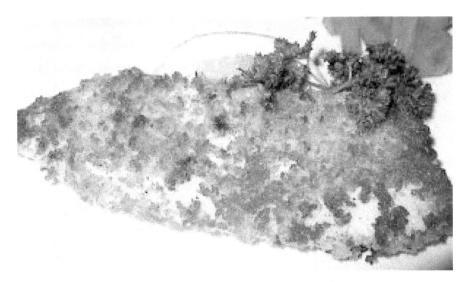

Cook Time: 5 minutes

Servings: 3

Ingredients:

2 tsp. Italian seasoning

2 tsp. lemon pepper

1/3 C. panko breadcrumbs

1/3 C. egg whites

1/3 C. almond flour

3 tilapia fillets

Olive oil

Directions:

Place panko, egg whites, and flour into separate bowls. Mix lemon pepper and Italian seasoning in with breadcrumbs.

Pat tilapia fillets dry. Dredge in flour, then egg, then breadcrumb mixture. Add to air fryer basket and spray lightly with olive oil.

Cook 10-11 minutes at 400 degrees, making sure to flip halfway through cooking.

Nutritional Values per serving: Calories: 256 Fat: 9g Protein: 39g Sugar: 5g

Air Fryer Pork Ribs

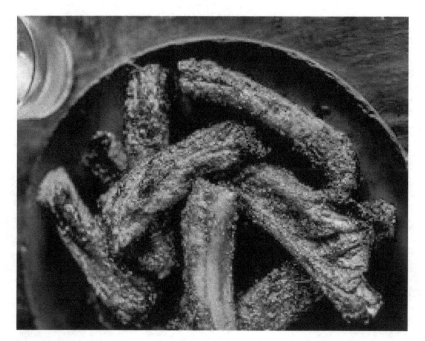

Cook Time: 27 minutes

Servings: 2

Ingredients:

1 lb. pork ribs

Salt and pepper to taste

½ cup BBQ sauce

1 teaspoon liquid Stevia

1 teaspoon spice mix

1 medium onion, chopped

1 tablespoon olive oil

Directions:

In a pan over medium heat, warm the oil. Add onion to pan and sauté for 2-minutes. Add spice mix, stevia, and BBQ sauce into pan and stir well. Remove pan from heat and set aside. Season pork ribs with salt and pepper and place inside of air fryer basket. Air fry the ribs at 320°Fahrenheit for 10-minutes. Brush BBQ sauce on both sides of pork. Air fry pork for an additional 15-minutes, cut into slices and serve.

Nutritional Values per serving: Calories: 284, Total Fat: 12.5g, Carbs: 11.2g, Protein: 16.5g

Vegetable Spring Rolls

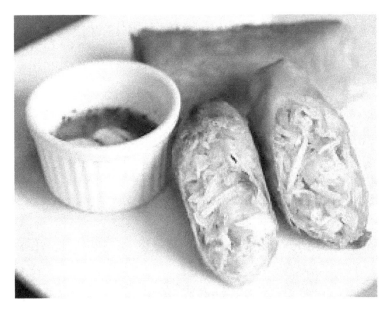

Cook Time: 23 minutes

Servings: 10

Ingredients:

10 spring roll wrappers

2 tablespoons cornstarch

Water

3 green onions, thinly sliced

1 tablespoon black pepper

1 teaspoon soy sauce

Pinches of salt

2 tablespoons cooking oil, plus more for brushing

8-cloves of garlic, minced

½ bell pepper, cut into thin matchsticks

2 large onions, cut into thin matchsticks

1 large carrot, cut into thin matchsticks

2 cups cabbage, shredded

2-inch piece of ginger, grated

Directions:

To prepare the filling: add to a large bowl the carrot, bell pepper, onion, cabbage, ginger, and garlic. Gently add two tablespoons of olive oil in a pan over high heat. Add the filling mixture and stir in salt and a dash of stevia sweetener if you like. Cook for 3-minutes. Add soy sauce, black pepper and mix well.

Add green onions, stir and set aside. In a small bowl, combine enough water and cornstarch to make a creamy paste. Fill the rolls with a tablespoon of filling in center of each wrapper and roll tightly, dampening the edges with cornstarch paste to ensure a good seal. Repeat until all wrappers and filling are used. Preheat your air fryer to 350°Fahrenheit. Brush the rolls with oil, and arrange them in the air fryer, and cook them until crisp and golden for about 20-minutes. Halfway through the cook time flip them over.

Nutritional Values per serving: Calories: 263, Total Fat: 11.2g, Carbs: 8.6g, Protein: 8.2g

Parsnip Fries

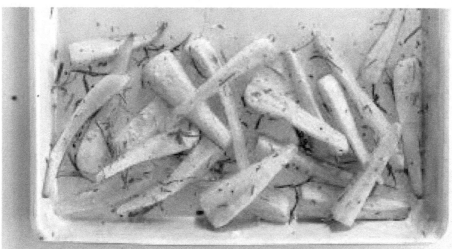

Cook Time: 12 minutes

Servings: 2

Ingredients:

2 tablespoons of olive oil

A pinch of sea salt

1 large bunch of parsnips

Directions:

Wash and peel the parsnips, then cut them into strips. Place the parsnips in a bowl with the olive oil and sea salt and coat well. Preheat your air fryer to 360°Fahrenheit. Place the parsnip and oil mixture into the air fryer basket. Cook for 12-minutes. Serve with sour cream or ketchup.

Nutritional Values per serving: Calories: 262g, Total Fat: 11.3g, Carbs: 10.4g, Protein: 7.2g

Bang Bang Panko Breaded Fried Shrimp

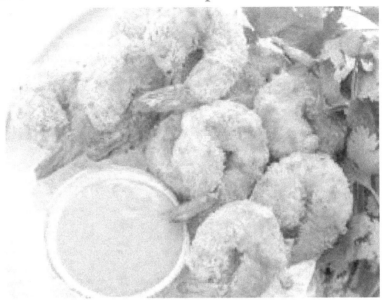

Cook Time: 15 minutes

Servings: 4

Ingredients:

1 tsp. paprika

Montreal chicken seasoning

¾ C. panko bread crumbs

½ C. almond flour

1 egg white

1 pound raw shrimp (peeled and deveined)

Bang Bang Sauce:

¼ C. sweet chili sauce

2 tbsp. sriracha sauce

1/3 C. plain Greek yogurt

Directions:

Ensure your air fryer is preheated to 400 degrees.

Season all shrimp with seasonings.

Add flour to one bowl, egg white in another, and breadcrumbs to a third.

Dip seasoned shrimp in flour, then egg whites, and then breadcrumbs.

Spray coated shrimp with olive oil and add to air fryer basket.

Cook 4 minutes, flip, and cook an additional 4 minutes.

To make the sauce, mix together all sauce ingredients until smooth.

Nutritional Values per serving: Calories: 212 Carbs: 12 Fat: 1g Protein: 37g Sugar: 0.5g

BBQ Pork Chops

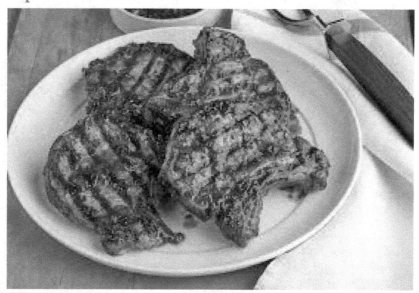

Cook Time: 10 minutes

Servings: 6

Ingredients:

6 pork loin chops

Pepper to taste

1 garlic clove

¼ teaspoon ground ginger

1 teaspoon balsamic vinegar

2 tablespoons soy sauce

2 tablespoons honey

Directions:

Preheat the air fryer to 350°Fahrenheit for 5-minutes. Season pork chops with pepper. In a mixing bowl, add soy sauce, honey, ground ginger, garlic, vinegar and mix well. Add seasoned pork chops to bowl and coat well. Place pork chops in fridge for 2 hours. Place marinated pork chops into air fryer basket and air fry for 10-minutes (5-minutes per side).

Nutritional Values per serving: Calories: 287, Total Fat: 12.4g, Carbs: 11.6g,

Ginger Garlic Pork Ribs

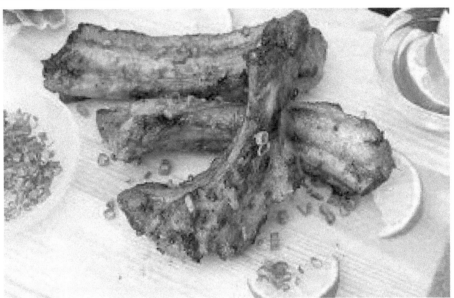

Cook Time: 40 minutes

Servings: 2

Ingredients:

1lb. baby pork ribs

1 tablespoon olive oil

1 tablespoon hoisin sauce

½ tablespoon honey

½ tablespoon soy sauce

3 garlic cloves, minced

Directions:

In a bowl, add the ingredients and mix well. Place the marinated ribs in fridge for 2-hours. Place marinated ribs in air fryer basket at 320°Fahrenheit for 40-minutes.

Nutritional Values per serving:, Calories: 287, Total Fat: 12.5g, Carbs: 11.5g, Protein: 16.2g

Bacon Wrapped Scallops

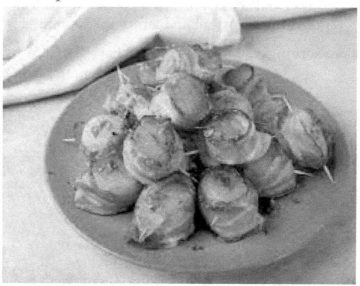

Cook Time: 10 minutes

Servings: 4

Ingredients:

1 tsp. paprika

1 tsp. lemon pepper

5 slices of center-cut bacon

20 raw sea scallops

Directions:

Rinse and drain scallops, placing on paper towels to soak up excess moisture.

Cut slices of bacon into 4 pieces.

Wrap each scallop with a piece of bacon, using toothpicks to secure. Sprinkle wrapped scallops with paprika and lemon pepper.

Spray air fryer basket with olive oil and add scallops.

Cook 5-6 minutes at 400 degrees, making sure to flip halfway through.

Nutritional Values per serving: Calories: 389 Fat: 17g Protein: 21g Sugar: 1g

Semolina Veggie Cutlets

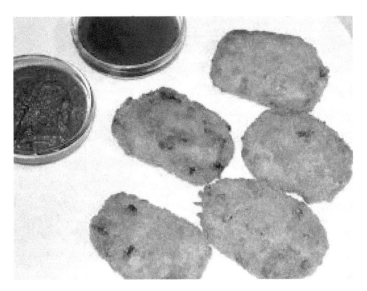

Cook Time: 23 minutes

Servings: 2

Ingredients:

1 cup semolina

Olive oil for frying

Salt and pepper to taste

1 ½ cups of your favorite veggies(suggestion: carrot, peas, green beans, bell pepper and cauliflower)

5 cups milk

Directions:

Stir and warm the milk in a saucepan over medium heat. Add vegetables when it becomes hot and cook until they are softened for about 3-minutes. Season with salt and pepper. Add the semolina to milk mixture and cook for another 10-minutes. Remove from heat and spread thin across a piece of parchment on a baking sheet, and chill for 4 hours in the fridge. Take out the baking sheet from the fridge, cut semolina mixture into cutlets. Preheat your air fryer to 350°Fahrenheit. Brush the cutlets with oil and bake for 10-minutes in your air fryer and serve with hot sauce!

Nutritional Value per serving: Calories: 252, Total Fat: 11.2g, Carbs: 10.3g, Protein: 7.3g

Perfect Cinnamon Toast

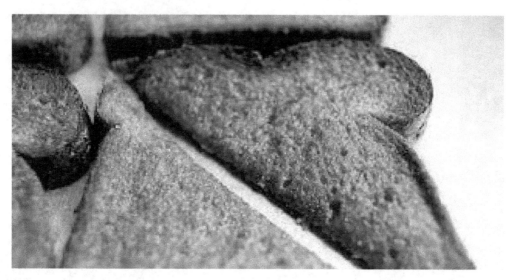

Cook Time: 5 minutes

Servings: 6

Ingredients:

2 tsp. pepper

1 ½ tsp. vanilla extract

1 ½ tsp. cinnamon

½ C. sweetener of choice

1 C. coconut oil

12 slices whole wheat bread

Directions:

Melt coconut oil and mix with sweetener until dissolved. Mix in remaining ingredients minus bread till incorporated.

Spread mixture onto bread, covering all area. Place coated pieces of bread in your air fryer.

Cook 5 minutes at 400 degrees.

Remove and cut diagonally. Enjoy!

Nutritional Values per serving: Calories: 124 Fat: 2g Protein: 0g Sugar: 4g

Chinese Pork Roast

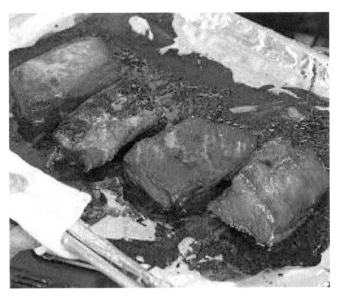

Cook Time: 15 minutes

Servings: 4

Ingredients:

2 lbs. pork shoulder, chopped

½ tablespoon salt

1/3 cup soy sauce

1 tablespoon honey

1 tablespoon liquid Stevia

Directions:

Place all the ingredients into a mixing bowl and combine well. Place marinated pork in fridge for 2-hours. Spray air fryer basket with cooking spray. Add marinated pork pieces into air fryer basket and cook at 350°Fahrenheit for 10-minutes. Now increase temperature to 400°Fahrenheit and cook for an additional 5-minutes.

Nutritional Values per serving: Calories: 283, Total Fat: 12.3g, Carbs: 11.5g, Protein: 16.7g

Air Fryer Salmon Patties

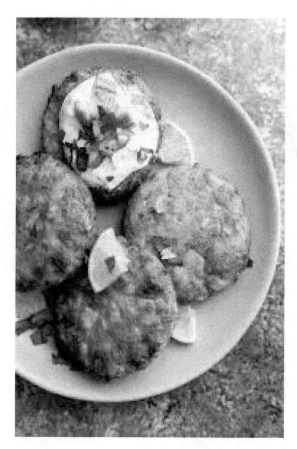

Cook Time: 15 minutes

Servings: 4

Ingredients:

1 tbsp. olive oil

1 tbsp. ghee

¼ tsp. salt

1/8 tsp. pepper

1 egg

1 C. almond flour

1 can wild Alaskan pink salmon

Directions:

Drain can of salmon into a bowl and keep liquid. Discard skin and bones.

Add salt, pepper, and egg to salmon, mixing well with hands to incorporate. Make patties.

Dredge in flour and remaining egg. If it seems dry, spoon reserved salmon liquid from the can onto patties.

Add patties to air fryer. Cook 7 minutes at 378 degrees till golden, making sure to flip once during cooking process.

Nutritional Values per serving: Calories: 437 Carbs: 55 Fat: 12g Protein: 24g Sugar: 2g

Fried Calamari

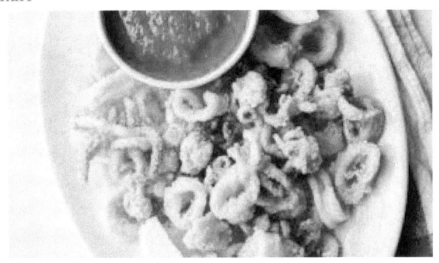

Cook Time: 15 minutes

Servings: 6-8

Ingredients:

½ tsp. salt

½ tsp. Old Bay seasoning

1/3 C. plain cornmeal

½ C. semolina flour

½ C. almond flour

5-6 C. olive oil

1 ½ pounds baby squid

Directions:

Rinse squid in cold water and slice tentacles, keeping just ¼-inch of the hood in one piece.

Combine 1-2 pinches of pepper, salt, Old Bay seasoning, cornmeal, and both flours together. Dredge squid pieces into flour mixture and place into air fryer. Spray liberally with olive oil.

Cook 15 minutes at 345 degrees till coating turns a golden brown.

Nutritional Values per serving: Calories: 211 Fat: 6g Protein: 21g Sugar: 1g

Crispy Air Fried Sushi Roll

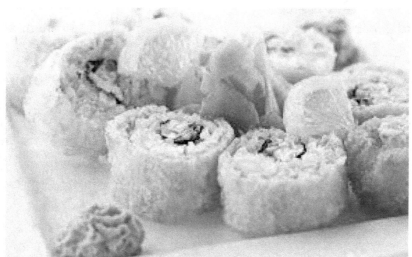

Cook Time: 15 minutes

Servings: 12

Ingredients:

Kale Salad:

1 tbsp. sesame seeds

¾ tsp. soy sauce

¼ tsp. ginger

1/8 tsp. garlic powder

¾ tsp. toasted sesame oil

½ tsp. rice vinegar

1 ½ C. chopped kale

Sriracha Mayo:

Sriracha sauce

¼ C. vegan mayo

 Coating:

½ C. panko breadcrumbs

Sushi Rolls:

½ of a sliced avocado

3 sheets of sushi nori

1 batch cauliflower rice

Directions:

Combine all of kale salad ingredients together, tossing well. Set to the side.

Lay out a sheet of nori and spread a handful of rice on. Then place 2-3 tbsp. of kale salad over rice, followed by avocado. Roll up sushi.

To make mayo, whisk mayo ingredients together until smooth.

Add breadcrumbs to a bowl. Coat sushi rolls in crumbs till coated and add to air fryer.

Cook rolls 10 minutes at 390 degrees, shaking gently at 5 minutes.

Slice each roll into 6-8 pieces and enjoy!

Nutritional Values per serving: Calories: 267 Fat: 13g Protein: 6g Sugar: 3g

Air Fryer Fish Tacos

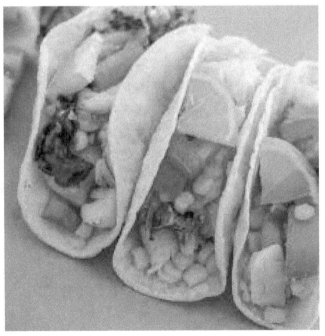

Cook Time: 5 minutes

Servings: 4

Ingredients:

1 pound cod

1 tbsp. cumin

½ tbsp. chili powder

1 ½ C. almond flour

1 ½ C. coconut flour

10 ounces Mexican beer

2 eggs

Directions:

Whisk beer and eggs together.

Whisk flours, pepper, salt, cumin, and chili powder together.
Slice cod into large pieces and coat in egg mixture then flour mixture.

Spray bottom of your air fryer basket with olive oil and add coated codpieces.

Cook 15 minutes at 375 degrees.

Serve on lettuce leaves topped with homemade salsa!

Nutritional Values per serving: Calories: 178 Fat: 10g Protein: 19g Sugar: 1g

Parmesan Shrimp

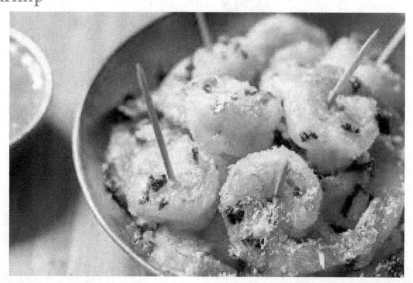

Cook Time: 10 minutes

Servings: 4-6

Ingredients:

2 tbsp. olive oil

1 tsp. onion powder

1 tsp. basil

½ tsp. oregano

1 tsp. pepper

2/3 C. grated parmesan cheese

4 minced garlic cloves

2 pounds of jumbo cooked shrimp (peeled/deveined)

Directions:

Mix all seasonings together and gently toss shrimp with mixture.

Spray olive oil into air fryer basket and add seasoned shrimp.

Cook 8-10 minutes at 350 degrees.

Squeeze lemon juice over shrimp right before devouring!

Nutritional Values per serving: Calories: 351 Fat: 11g Protein: 19g Sugar: 1g

Honey Glazed Salmon

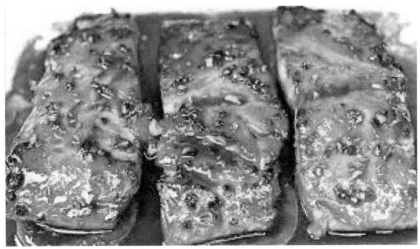

Cook Time: 5 minutes

Servings: 2

Ingredients:

1 tsp. water

3 tsp. rice wine vinegar

6 tbsp. low-sodium soy sauce

6 tbsp. raw honey

2 salmon fillets

Directions:

Combine water, vinegar, honey, and soy sauce together. Pour half of this mixture into a bowl.

Place salmon in one bowl of marinade and let chill 2 hours.

Ensure your air fryer is preheated to 356 degrees and add salmon.

Cook 8 minutes, flipping halfway through. Baste salmon with some of the remaining marinade mixture and cook another 5 minutes.

To make a sauce to serve salmon with, pour remaining marinade mixture into a saucepan, heating till simmering. Let simmer 2 minutes. Serve drizzled over salmon!

Nutritional Values per serving: Calories: 390 Fat: 8g Protein: 16g Sugar: 5g

Apple Dumplings

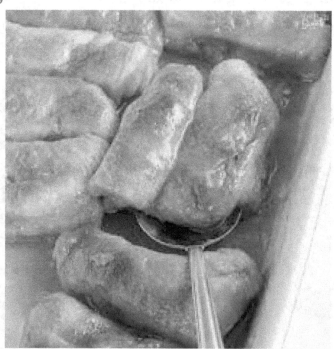

Cook Time: 15 minutes

Servings: 4

Ingredients:

2 tbsp. melted coconut oil

2 puff pastry sheets

1 tbsp. brown sugar

2 tbsp. raisins

2 small apples of choice

Directions:

Ensure your air fryer is preheated to 356 degrees.

Core and peel apples and mix with raisins and sugar.

Place a bit of apple mixture into puff pastry sheets and brush sides with melted coconut oil.

Place into air fryer. Cook 25 minutes, turning halfway through. Will be golden when done.

Nutritional Values per serving: Calories: 367 Fat: 7g Protein: 2g Sugar: 5g

Chapter 5: Dinner

Crumbed Pork & Semi-Dried Tomato Pesto

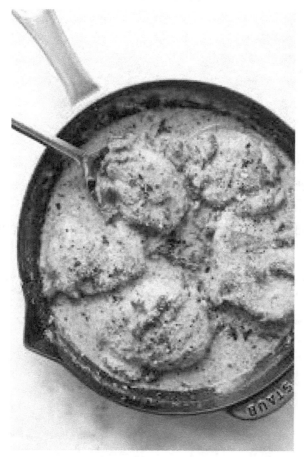

Cook Time: 20 minutes

Servings: 2

Ingredients:

½ cup milk

1 egg

1 cup breadcrumbs

1 tablespoon parmesan cheese, grated

¼ bunch of thyme, chopped

1 teaspoon pine nuts

¼ cup semi-dried tomatoes

½ cup almond flour

2 pork cutlets

1 lemon, zested

Sea salt and black pepper to taste

6 basil leaves

1 tablespoon olive oil

Directions:

Combine and whisk milk and egg in a bowl, then set aside. Mix in another bowl, breadcrumbs, parmesan, thyme, lemon zest, salt, and pepper. Add flour to another bowl. Dip pork cutlet in flour, then into egg and milk mixture, and finally into breadcrumb mixture. Preheat air fryer to 360°Fahrenheit. Spray basket with cooking spray. Set the air fryer timer to 20-minutes. Place pork inside of basket and cook until golden and crisp. Prepare the pesto: add the tomatoes, pine nuts, olive oil, and basil leaves into food processor. Blend for 20-seconds. When the pork is ready, serve with pesto and a salad of your choice.

Nutritional Values per serving: Calories: 264, Total Fat: 13.2g, Carbs: 11.7g, Protein: 16.3g

Pork Loin with Potatoes & Herbs

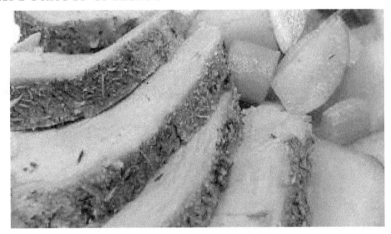

Cook Time: 25 minutes

Servings: 2

Ingredients:

2 lbs. pork loin

½ teaspoon garlic powder

½ teaspoon red pepper flakes

½ teaspoon black pepper

2 large potatoes, chunked

Directions:

Sprinkle the pork loin with garlic powder, red pepper flakes, parsley, salt, and pepper. Preheat your air fryer to 370°Fahrenheit and place pork loin and potatoes to one side in basket of air fryer. Cook for 25-minutes. Remove the pork loin and potatoes from air fryer. Allow pork loin to cool before slicing and enjoy!

Nutritional Values per serving: Calories: 268, Total Fat: 12.3g, Carbs: 11.6g, Protein: 16.2g

Tasty Beef Burgers

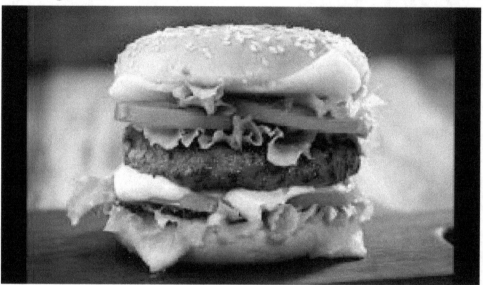

Cook Time: 18 minutes

Servings: 4

Ingredients:

1 ½ lbs. ground beef

1 tablespoon Montreal steak seasoning

1 cup cheddar cheese, shredded

1 tablespoon Worcestershire sauce

½ cup cheese sauce

Directions:

Preheat your air fryer to 370°Fahrenheit. Add the ground beef, Montreal steak seasoning, Worcestershire sauce in a bowl and mix well. Make four patties from mixture and place in preheated air fryer basket and cook for 15-minutes. Flip the patties halfway through.

Combine the cheese sauce and cheddar cheese. Add cheese mixture to the top of patties and cook for an additional 3-minutes. Serve warm!

Nutritional Values per serving: Calories: 302, Total Fat: 12.3g, Carbs: 11.2g, Protein: 16.4g

Chinese Pork Ribs

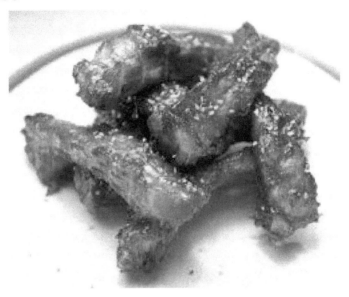

Cook Time: 40 minutes

Servings: 6

Ingredients:

4 garlic cloves, minced

1 tablespoon honey

2 lbs. pork ribs

2 tablespoons sesame oil

2 tablespoons ginger, minced

2 tablespoons hoisin sauce

2 tablespoons char Siu sauce

1 tablespoon soy sauce

Directions:

Place the ingredients in a bowl except for meat and combine well. Place the ribs in a bowl and pour the sauce over them and coat well. Place in the fridge for 4-hours. Place ribs into air fryer at 330°Fahrenheit for 40-minutes. Increase the temperature of air fryer to 350°Fahrenheit and cook for an additional 10-minutes. Serve warm.

Nutritional Values per serving: Calories: 287, Total Fat: 12.3g, Carbs: 10.6g, Protein: 16.2g

Turkey Sausage Patties

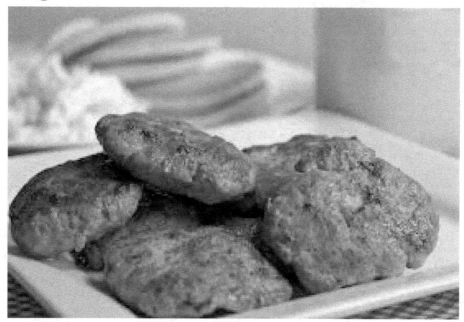

Cook Time: 4 minutes

Servings: 6

Ingredients:

1 teaspoon olive oil

1 small onion, diced

1 large garlic clove, chopped

Salt and pepper to taste

1 tablespoon vinegar

1 tablespoon chives, chopped

¾ teaspoon paprika

Pinch of nutmeg

1 lb. lean ground turkey

1 teaspoon fennel seeds

Directions:

Preheat your air fryer to 375°Fahrenheit. Add half of the oil along with onion and garlic to air fryer. Air fry for 1-minute then add fennel seeds then transfer to plate. In a mixing bowl, mix paprika, ground turkey, nutmeg, chives, vinegar, salt pepper, and onion. Mix well and form patties. Add the remaining oil to your air fryer and air fry patties for 3-minutes. Serve on buns.

Nutritional Values per serving: Calories: 302, Total Fat: 12.2g, Carbs: 10.2g, Protein: 16.3g

Pork Satay with Peanut Sauce

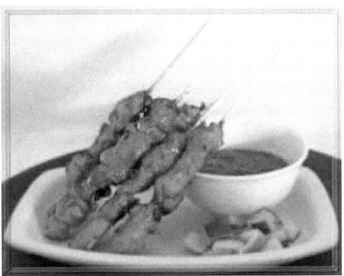

Cook Time: 21 minutes

Servings: 4

Ingredients:

1 teaspoon ground ginger

2 teaspoons hot pepper sauce

2 cloves garlic, crushed

3 tablespoons sweet soy sauce

3 ½ ounces unsalted peanuts, ground

¾ cup coconut milk

1 teaspoon ground coriander

2 tablespoons vegetable oil

14-ounces lean pork chops, in cubes of 1-inch

Directions:

In a large mixing bowl, combine hot sauce, ginger, half garlic, oil and soy sauce. Place the meat into the mixture and leave for 15-minutes to marinate. Place the meat into wire basket of your air fryer. Cook at 390°Fahrenheit for 12-minutes. Turn over halfway through cook time. For the peanut sauce, place the oil into a skillet and heat it up. Add the garlic and coriander and cook for 5-minutes, stirring often. Add the coconut milk, peanuts, hot pepper sauce and soy sauce to the pan and bring to boil. Stir often. Remove the pork from air fryer and pour sauce over it and serve warm.

Nutritional Values per serving: Calories: 262, Total Fat: 12.3g, Carbs: 11.4g, Protein: 17.3g

Onion Carrot Meatloaf

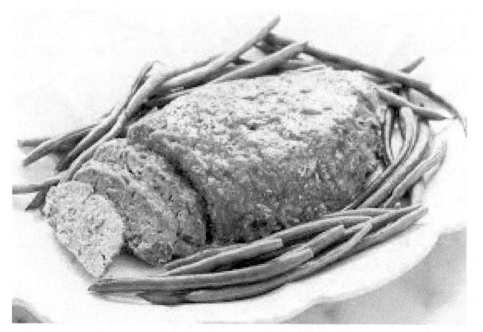

Cook Time: 25 minutes

Servings: 6

Ingredients:

1 lb. ground beef

Salt and pepper to taste

½ cup breadcrumbs

¼ cup milk

½ onion, shredded

2 carrots, shredded

1 egg

Directions:

Preheat your air fryer to 400°Fahrenheit. Mix all your ingredients in a bowl. Add the meatloaf mixture to a loaf pan and place it in your air fryer basket. Cook in air fryer for 25-minutes and serve warm.

Nutritional Values per serving: Calories: 306, Total Fat: 12.7g, Carbs: 12.3g, Protein: 16.8g

Mozzarella Turkey Rolls

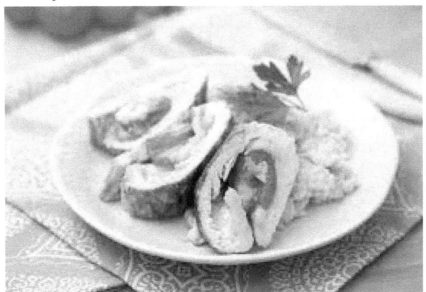

Cook Time: 10 minutes

Servings: 4

Ingredients:

4 slices turkey breast

4 chive shoots (for tying rolls)

1 tomato, sliced

½ cup basil, fresh, chopped

1 cup mozzarella, sliced

Directions:

Preheat your air fryer to 390°Fahrenheit. Place the slices of mozzarella cheese, tomato, and basil onto each slice of turkey. Roll up and tie with chive shoot. Place into air fryer and cook for 10-minutes. Serve warm.

Nutritional Values per serving: Calories: 296, Total Fat: 12.4g, Carbs: 10.2g, Protein: 16.2g

Turkey Balls Stuffed with Sage & Onion

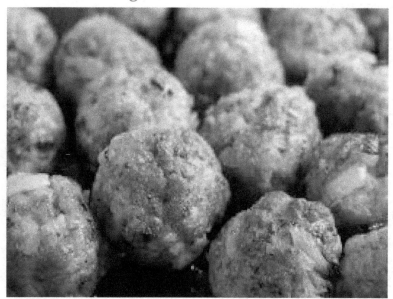

Cook Time: 15 minutes

Servings: 2

Ingredients:

3.5 ounces ground turkey

3 tablespoons breadcrumbs

Salt and pepper to taste

1 teaspoon sage

½ small onion, diced

1 egg

Directions:

Add all the ingredients into large mixing bowl and combine well. Form the mixture into small balls and put in air fryer and cook at 350°Fahrenheit for 15-minutes. Serve with tartar sauce and mashed potatoes.

Nutritional Values per serving: Calories: 268, Total Fat: 9.8g, Carbs: 8.6g, Protein: 11.9g

Chicken Schnitzel

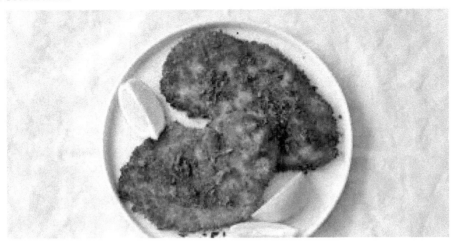

Cook Time: 12 minutes

Servings: 4

Ingredients:

2 chicken breasts

Salt and pepper to taste

Fresh parsley

2 tablespoons mustard powder

12 tablespoons gluten-free oats

2 free-range eggs

Directions:

Slice your chicken breasts into two lengthwise and use a rolling pin to roll them flat. Sprinkle with salt and pepper and then set aside. In a small bowl whisk the eggs and set aside. In your blender grind the oats with mustard, salt, pepper, and parsley. You want it to become like breadcrumbs. Place this mixture into a shallow dish. Dip chicken pieces into the egg and coat well. Next, dip them into the oats breadcrumb mixture. Place chicken pieces in your air fryer and cook for 12-minutes at 350°Fahrenheit. Flip over the chicken pieces halfway through the cook time.

Nutritional Values per serving: Calories: 282, Total Fat: 10.2g, Carbs: 8.7g, Protein: 14.8g

Turkey & Cheese Calzone

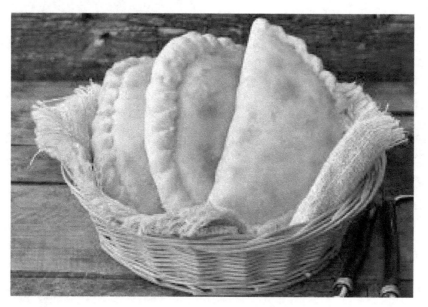

Cook Time: 10 minutes

Servings: 4

Ingredients:

1 free-range egg, beaten

¼ cup mozzarella cheese, grated

1 cup cheddar cheese, grated

1-ounce bacon, diced, cooked

Cooked turkey, shredded

4 tablespoons tomato sauce

Salt and pepper to taste

1 teaspoon thyme

1 teaspoon basil

1 teaspoon oregano

1 package frozen pizza dough

Directions:

Roll the pizza dough out into small circles, the same size as a small pizza. Add thyme, oregano, basil into a bowl with tomato sauce and mix well. Pour a small amount of sauce onto your pizza bases and spread across the surface. Add the turkey, bacon, and cheese. Brush the edge of dough with beaten egg, then fold over and pinch to seal. Brush the outside with more egg. Place into air fryer and cook at 350°Fahrenehit for 10-minutes. Serve warm.

Nutritional Values per serving: Calories: 289, Total Fat: 11.2g, Carbs: 10.3g, Protein: 11.4g

Country Style Ribs

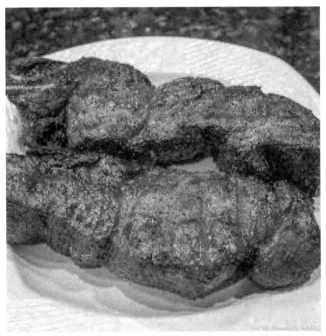

Cook Time: 12 minutes

Servings: 4

Ingredients:

4 country-style pork ribs, trimmed of excess fat

Salt and black pepper to taste

1 teaspoon dried marjoram

1 teaspoon garlic powder

1 teaspoon thyme

2 teaspoons dry mustard

3 tablespoons coconut oil

3 tablespoons cornstarch

Directions:

Preheat the air fryer to 400°Fahrenheit for 2 minutes. Place ingredients in a bowl, except pork ribs. Soak the ribs in the mixture and rub in. Place the ribs into air fryer for 12-minutes. Serve and enjoy!

Nutritional Value per serving: Calories: 265, Total Fat: 12.6g, Carbs: 12.2g, Protein: 16.5g

Air Fryer Classic Beef Pot Roast

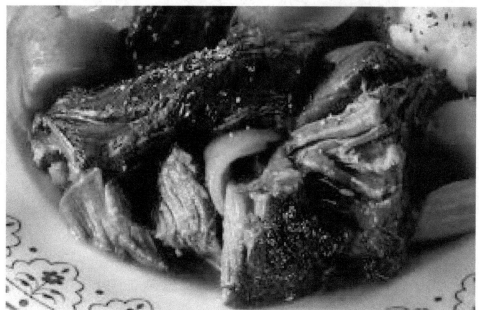

Cook Time: 60 minutes

Servings: 4

Ingredients:

1 lb. chuck roast

4 spring onions

2 cinnamon sticks

2 tablespoons of ginger garlic paste

2 tablespoons of olive oil

1 teaspoon paprika

2 cardamoms

1 cup of water

½ cup of fresh coriander, chopped

Salt and pepper to taste

1 bay leaf

Directions:

Preheat your air fryer to 400°Fahrenheit. Cut the chuck roast into medium-sized chunks. In a large bowl, add beef, onion, ginger garlic paste, salt, pepper, bay leaf, coriander, cardamoms, paprika, and water. Mix well and marinate for 1-hour. Add everything to casserole dish and roast in the air fryer for 1-hour. Remove bay leaf then serve hot!

Nutritional Values per serving: Calories: 303, Total Fat: 12.6g, Carbs: 11.3g, Protein: 16.4g

Sweet & Tangy Meatballs

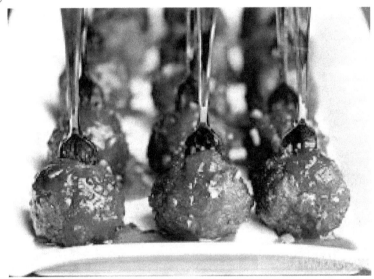

Cook Time: 15 minutes

Servings: 24

Ingredients:

1 lb. ground beef

1 tablespoon liquid stevia

½ teaspoon dry mustard

½ teaspoon ginger, ground

¾ cup tomato ketchup

1 tablespoon Tabasco sauce

1 tablespoon Worcestershire sauce

¼ cup vinegar

1 tablespoon lemon juice

Directions:

In a bowl, combine all the ingredients. Make small meatballs from the mixture and place them in air fryer basket. Air fry meatballs at 370°Fahrenheit for 15-minutes. Serve warm.

Nutritional Values per serving: Calories: 298, Total Fat: 12.2g, Carbs: 11.6g, Protein: 15.8g

Cheese Burgers

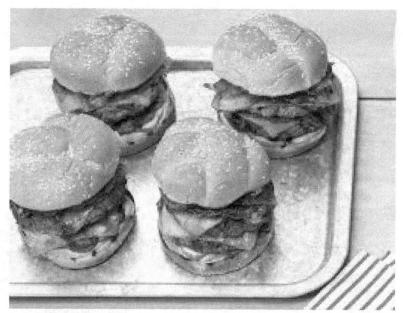

Cook Time: 11 minutes

Servings: 6

Ingredients:

1 lb. ground beef

6 slices cheddar cheese

Salt and pepper to taste

Directions:

Preheat the air fryer to 350°Fahrenheit. Season ground beef with pepper and salt. Make six patties from the mixture and place them into air fryer basket. Air fry patties for 10-minutes. After 10-minutes, place cheese slices over patties and cook for another minute. Serve warm.

Nutritional Values per serving: Calories: 302, Total Fat: 12.5g, Carbs: 12.2g, Protein: 16.2g

Air Fryer Beef Fajitas

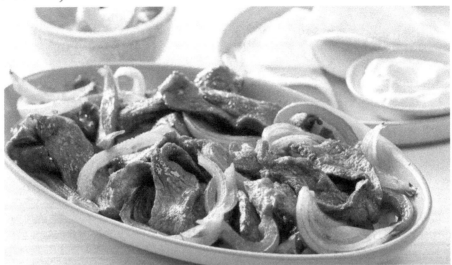

Calories: 412 Fat: 21g Protein: 13g Sugar: 1g

Cook Time: 5 minutes

Servings: 4-6

Ingredients:

Beef:

- 1/8 C. carne asada seasoning
- 2 pounds beef flap meat
- Diet 7-Up

Fajita veggies:

- 1 tsp. chili powder
- 1-2 tsp. pepper
- 1-2 tsp. salt
- 2 bell peppers, your choice of color
- 1 onion

Directions:

- Slice flap meat into manageable pieces and place into a bowl. Season meat with carne seasoning and pour diet soda over meat. Cover and chill overnight.
- Ensure your air fryer is preheated to 380 degrees.

- Place a parchment liner into air fryer basket and spray with olive oil. Place beef in layers into the basket.
- Cook 8-10 minutes, making sure to flip halfway through. Remove and set to the side.
- Slice up veggies and spray air fryer basket. Add veggies to the fryer and spray with olive oil. Cook 10 minutes at 400 degrees, shaking 1-2 times during cooking process.
- Serve meat and veggies on wheat tortillas and top with favorite keto fillings!

Turkey Breast with Maple Mustard Glaze

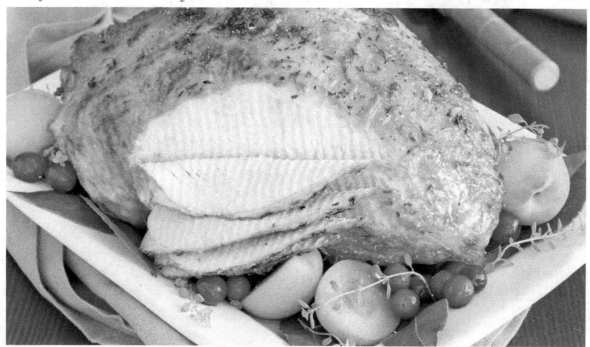

Cook Time: 49 minutes

Servings: 6

Ingredients:

5 lbs. turkey breast

1 tablespoon unsalted butter

2 tablespoons Dijon mustard

¼ cup sugar-free maple syrup

½ teaspoon black pepper

1 teaspoon sea salt

½ teaspoon paprika

1 teaspoon dried thyme

1 tablespoon olive oil

½ teaspoon sage

Directions:

Preheat your air fryer to 350°Fahrenheit. Prepare the turkey breast by brushing it with olive oil. Combine salt, pepper, paprika, sage, thyme in a bowl. Cover the turkey breast with this mixture. Place the turkey breast inside air fryer and cook for 25-minutes. Turn and cook for another 12-minutes. Turn once more and cook for an additional 12-minutes. Use a small saucepan to mix mustard, melted butter, and maple syrup, stir well. When turkey breast is done cooking, cover with sauce. Then air-fry for another 5-minutes. Take the turkey out of air fryer and set aside for at least 5-minutes, covering with aluminum foil. Slice turkey and serve.

Nutritional Values per serving: Calories: 268, Total Fat: 10.2g, Carbs: 8.5g, Protein: 14.3g

Beef Empanadas

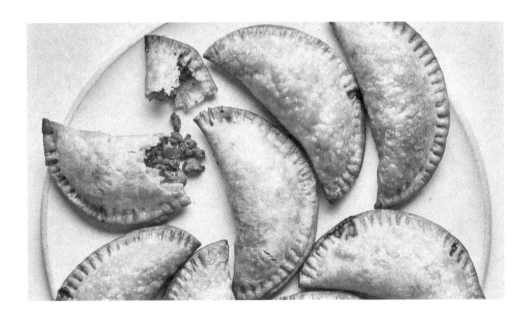

Calories: 183 Fat: 5g Protein: 11g Sugar: 2g

Cook Time: 15 minutes

Servings: 8

Ingredients:

- 1 tsp. water
- 1 egg white
- 1 C. picadillo
- 8 Goya empanada discs (thawed)

Directions:

- Ensure your air fryer is preheated to 325. Spray basket with olive oil.
- Place 2 tablespoons of picadillo into the center of each disc. Fold disc in half and use a fork to seal edges. Repeat with all ingredients.
- Whisk egg white with water and brush tops of empanadas with egg wash.
- Add 2-3 empanadas to air fryer, cooking 8 minutes until golden. Repeat till you cook all filled empanadas.

Air Fryer Burgers

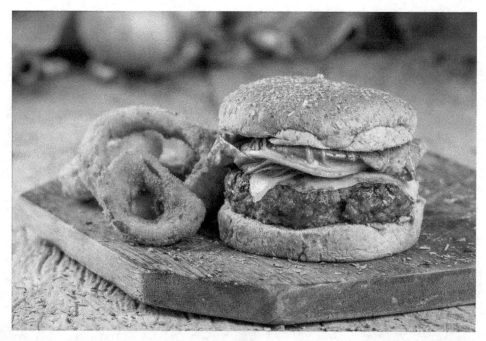

Calories: 148 Fat: 5g Protein: 24g Sugar: 1g

Cook Time: 10 minutes

Servings: 4

Ingredients:

- 1 pound lean ground beef
- ½ tsp. garlic powder
- ½ tsp. dried oregano
- ½ tsp. pepper
- ½ tsp. salt
- ½ tsp. onion powder
- Few drops of liquid smoke
- 1 tsp. Worcestershire sauce
- 1 tsp. dried parsley

Directions:

- Ensure your air fryer is preheated to 350 degrees.
- Mix all seasonings together till combined.
- Place beef in a bowl and add seasonings. Mix well, but do not overmix.
- Make 4 patties from the mixture and using your thumb, making an indent in the center of each patty.
- Add patties to air fryer basket and cook 10 minutes. No need to turn!

Roasted Stuffed Peppers

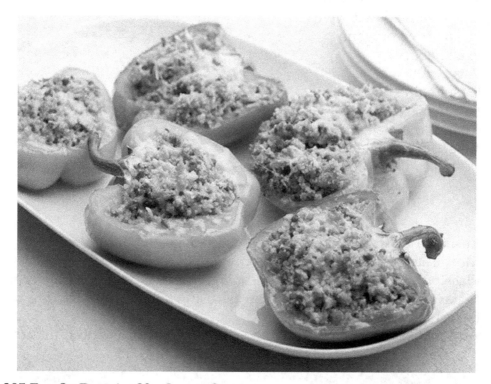

Calories: 295 Fat: 8g Protein: 23g Sugar: 2g

Cook Time: 5 minutes

Servings: 4

Ingredients:

- 4 ounces shredded cheddar cheese
- ½ tsp. pepper
- ½ tsp. salt
- 1 tsp. Worcestershire sauce
- ½ C. tomato sauce
- 8 ounces lean ground beef
- 1 tsp. olive oil
- 1 minced garlic clove
- ½ chopped onion
- 2 green peppers

Directions:

- Ensure your air fryer is preheated to 390 degrees. Spray with olive oil.
- Cut stems off bell peppers and remove seeds. Cook in boiling salted water for 3 minutes.
- Sauté garlic and onion together in a skillet until golden in color.
- Take skillet off the heat. Mix pepper, salt, Worcestershire sauce, ¼ cup of tomato sauce, half of cheese and beef together.
- Divide meat mixture into pepper halves. Top filled peppers with remaining cheese and tomato sauce.
- Place filled peppers in air fryer and bake 15-20 minutes.

Air Fryer Beef Steak

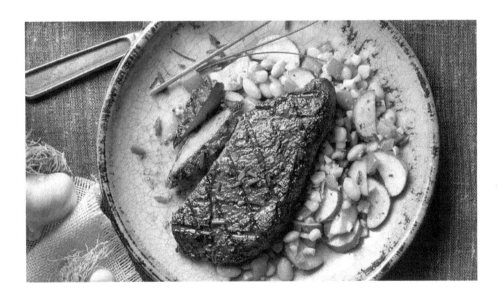

Calories: 233 Fat: 19g Protein: 16g Sugar: 0g

Cook Time: 17 minutes

Servings: 4

Ingredients:

- 1 tbsp. olive oil
- Pepper and salt
- 2 pounds of ribeye steak

Directions:

- Season meat on both sides with pepper and salt.
- Rub all sides of meat with olive oil.
- Preheat air fryer to 356 degrees and spritz with olive oil.
- Cook steak 7 minutes. Flip and cook an additional 6 minutes.
- Let meat sit 2-5 minutes to rest. Slice and serve with salad.

Beef and Broccoli

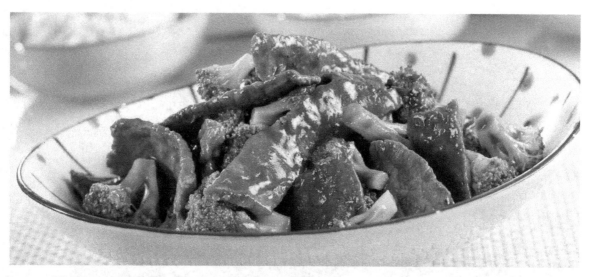

Calories: 384 Fat: 16g Protein: 19g Sugar: 4g

Cook Time: 10 minutes

Servings: 4

Ingredients:

- 1 minced garlic clove
- 1 sliced ginger root
- 1 tbsp. olive oil
- 1 tsp. almond flour
- 1 tsp. sweetener of choice
- 1 tsp. low-sodium soy sauce

- 1/3 C. sherry
- 2 tsp. sesame oil
- 1/3 C. oyster sauce
- 1 pounds of broccoli
- ¾ pound round steak

Directions:

- Remove stems from broccoli and slice into florets. Slice steak into thin strips.
- Combine sweetener, soy sauce, sherry, almond flour, sesame oil, and oyster sauce together, stirring till sweetener dissolves.
- Put strips of steak into the mixture and allow to marinate 45 minutes to 2 hours.
- Add broccoli and marinated steak to air fryer. Place garlic, ginger, and olive oil on top.
- Cook 12 minutes at 400 degrees. Serve with cauliflower rice!

Coconut Shrimp

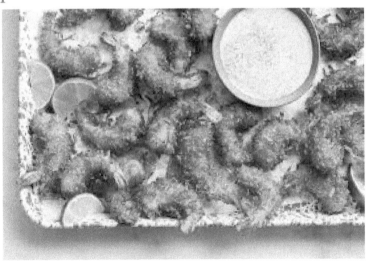

Calories: 213 Fat: 8g Protein: 15g Sugar: 3g

Cook Time: 5 minutes

Servings: 3

Ingredients:

- 1 C. almond flour
- 1 C. panko breadcrumbs

- 1 tbsp. coconut flour
- 1 C. unsweetened, dried coconut
- 1 egg white
- 12 raw large shrimp

Directions:

- Put shrimp on paper towels to drain.
- Mix coconut and panko breadcrumbs together. Then mix in coconut flour and almond flour in a different bowl. Set to the side.
- Dip shrimp into flour mixture, then into egg white, and then into coconut mixture.
- Place into air fryer basket. Repeat with remaining shrimp.
- Cook 10 minutes at 350 degrees. Turn halfway through cooking process.

Air Fryer Salmon

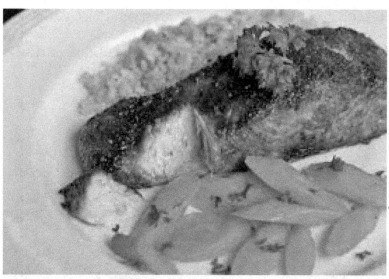

Calories: 185 Fat: 11g Protein: 21g Sugar: 0g

Cook Time: 5 minutes

Servings: 2

Ingredients:

- ½ tsp. salt
- ½ tsp. garlic powder
- ½ tsp. smoked paprika
- Salmon

Directions:

- Mix spices together and sprinkle onto salmon.
- Place seasoned salmon into air fryer.
- Cook 8-10 minutes at 400 degrees.

Healthy Fish and Chips

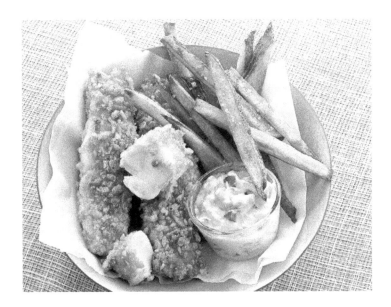

Calories: 219 Carbs: 18 Fat: 5g Protein: 25g Sugar: 1g

Cook Time: 15 minutes

Servings: 3

Ingredients:

- Old Bay seasoning
- ½ C. panko breadcrumbs
- 1 egg
- 2 tbsp. almond flour
- 2 4-6 ounce tilapia fillets
- Frozen crinkle cut fries

Directions:

- Add almond flour to one bowl, beat egg in another bowl, and add panko breadcrumbs to the third bowl, mixed with Old Bay seasoning.

- Dredge tilapia in flour, then egg, and then breadcrumbs.
- Place coated fish in air fryer along with fries.
- Cook 15 minutes at 390 degrees.

Chapter 6: Appetizers & Side Dishes

Spanish Style Spiced Potatoes

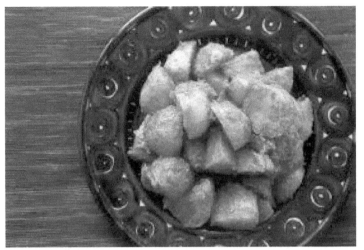

Cook Time: 23 minutes

Servings: 4

Ingredients:

3 potatoes, peeled and chopped into chips

1 onion, diced

½ cup tomato sauce

1 tomato, thinly sliced

1 tablespoon red wine vinegar

2 tablespoons olive oil

1 teaspoon paprika

1 teaspoon chili powder

Salt and pepper to taste

1 teaspoon rosemary

1 teaspoon oregano

1 teaspoon mixed spice

2 teaspoons coriander

Directions:

Toss the chips in the olive oil and cook in your air fryer for 15-minutes at 360°Fahrenheit. Mix remaining ingredients in a baking dish. Place the sauce in air fryer for 8-minutes. Toss the potatoes in the sauce and serve warm!

Nutritional Values per serving: Calories: 265, Total Fat: 7,3g, Carbs: 6.2g, Protein: 5.2g

Bell Peppers with Potato Stuffing

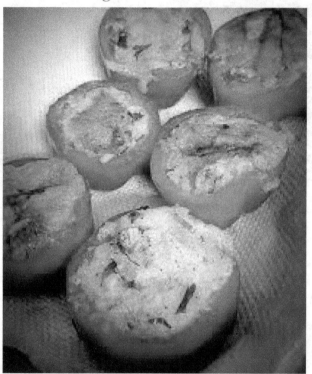

Cook Time: 20 minutes

Servings: 4

Ingredients:

4 green bell peppers, top cut and deseeded

4 potatoes, boiled, peeled and mashed

2 onions, finely chopped

1 teaspoon lemon juice

2 tablespoons coriander leaves, chopped

2 green chilies, finely chopped

Olive oil as needed

Salt to taste

¼ teaspoon Garam Masala

½ teaspoon chili powder

¼ teaspoon turmeric powder

1 teaspoon cumin seeds

Directions:

Heat the oil in a pan and sauté the onion, chilies and cumin seeds. Add the rest of the ingredients except the bell peppers and mix well. Preheat your air fryer to 390°Fahrenheit for 10-minutes. Brush your bell peppers with olive oil, inside and out and stuff each pepper with potato mixture. Place in air fryer basket and grill for 10-minutes. Check and grill for an additional 5-minutes.

Nutritional Values per serving: Calories: 282, Total Fat: 9.2g, Carbs: 7.1g, Protein: 4.2g

Chopped Liver with Eggs

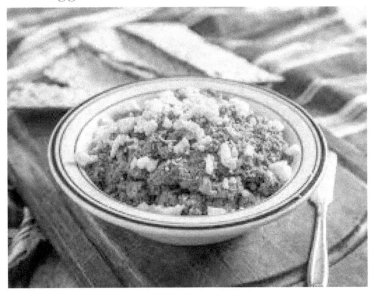

Cook Time: 12 minutes

Servings: 2

Ingredients:

2 large eggs

1 lb. sliced liver

Salt and pepper to taste

1 tablespoon cream

½ tablespoon black truffle oil

1 tablespoon butter

Directions:

Preheat your air fryer to 340°Fahrenheit. Cut liver into thin slices and place in the fridge. Separate the whites from the yolks of the eggs and put each yolk in a cup. In another bowl, add the cream, the black truffle oil, salt, pepper and beat to combine. Take the liver and arrange half of the mixture in a small ramekin. Pour the white of the egg and divide equally between two ramekins. Put the yolks on top. Surround the yolks with the liver and cook for 12-minutes. Serve cool.

Nutritional Values per serving: Calories: 374, Total Fat: 10g, Carbs: 8.5g, Protein: 59g

Bacon & Veggie Mash

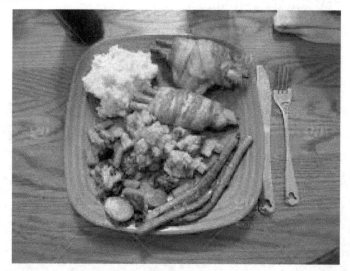

Cook Time: 1 hour and 15 minutes

Servings: 8

Ingredients:

4 strips of bacon, chopped into pieces

1 tablespoon butter

¾ cup Yellow onion, diced

½ cup red bell pepper, diced

¼ cup celery, diced

2 teaspoons garlic, minced

¾ teaspoon fresh thyme leaves

1 ½ cups whole milk

3 eggs

½ cup heavy cream

1 teaspoon sea salt

¼ teaspoon cayenne pepper

3 cups day-old bread, cubed

3 tablespoons parmesan cheese, grated

1 cup Monterey Jack cheese grated

Seasoning:

2 ½ teaspoons paprika

2 teaspoons salt

2 teaspoons garlic powder

1 teaspoon black pepper

1 teaspoon onion powder

1 teaspoon cayenne pepper

1 teaspoon oregano, dried

1 teaspoon thyme, dried

Directions:

Grease a casserole dish with the butter. Cook bacon in small frying pan until crisp, then place aside. Cook the corn in the pan until caramelized for about 10-minutes, then add in celery, onion, bell pepper and cook for an additional 5-minutes. Mix in the thyme and garlic and remove from heat. Stir in the eggs, milk, and cream, whisking well to combine. Add in salt, cayenne pepper, bread and Monterey Jack cheese. Transfer to casserole dish and place in air fryer basket. Cook for 30-minutes at 320°Fahrenheit. Sprinkle with parmesan cheese and cook for another 30-minutes.

Nutritional Values per serving: Calories: 42, Total Fat: 8.3g, Carbs: 9.5g, Protein: 16.2g

Spicy Cheesy Breaded Mushrooms

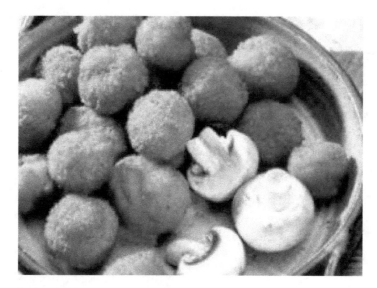

Cook Time: 7 minutes

Servings: 2

Ingredients:

8-ounces of Button mushrooms (pat dried)

1 egg

Almond flour as required

3-ounces parmesan cheese, freshly grated

Breadcrumbs as needed

Salt and pepper to taste

1 teaspoon paprika

Directions:

Mix the cheese and the breadcrumbs and paprika in a mixing bowl. Whisk the egg in another bowl. Dredge the Button mushrooms in the flour, dip in egg then coat them in breadcrumb mix. Cook for 7-minutes in your air fryer at 360° Fahrenheit, tossing once halfway through cook time.

Nutritional Values per serving: Calories: 203, Total Fat: 4.2g, Carbs: 3.2g, Protein: 3.6g

Chickpea & Zucchini Burgers

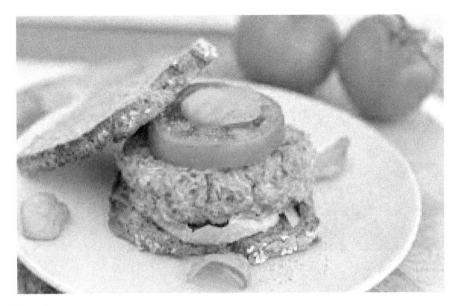

Cook Time: 10 minutes

Servings: 4

Ingredients:

1 can of chickpeas, strained

1 red onion, diced

2 eggs, beaten

1-ounce almond flour

3 tablespoons coriander

1 teaspoon garlic puree

1-ounce cheddar cheese, shredded

1 Courgette, spiralized

1 teaspoon chili powder

Salt and pepper to taste

1 teaspoon mixed spice

Directions:

Add your ingredients to a bowl and mix well. Shape portions of the mixture into burgers. Place in the air fryer for 15-minutes until cooked.

Nutritional Values per serving: Calories: 263, Total Fat: 11.2g, Carbs: 8.3g, Protein: 6.3g

Turmeric & Garlic Roasted Carrots

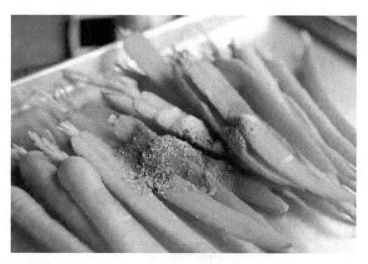

Cook Time: 20 minutes

Servings: 4

Ingredients:

21-ounces of carrots, peeled

1 handful of fresh coriander

1 teaspoon turmeric

1 tablespoon olive oil

1 teaspoon garlic, minced

Directions:

Lightly drizzle the olive oil over the carrots and sprinkle the turmeric and garlic over them. Place in pan in air fryer and cook for 20-minutes at 290°Fahrenheit. Toss once during cook time. Serve carrots garnished with fresh coriander.

Nutritional Values per serving: Calories: 60, Total Fat: 0.35g, Carbs: 10.2g, Protein: 0.48g

Vegetable Fries

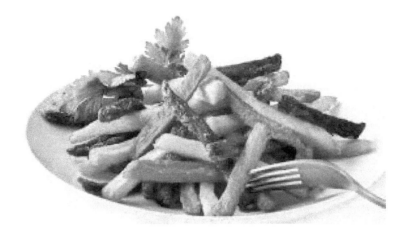

Cook Time: 18 minutes

Servings: 4

Ingredients:

5-ounces sweet potatoes, peeled and chopped as chips

5-ounces Courgette, peeled and chopped as chips

5-ounces carrots, peeled and chopped as chips

2 tablespoons olive oil

Salt and pepper to taste

Pinch of basil

Pinch of mixed spice

Directions:

Toss the veggies in olive oil and place in an air fryer preheated to 360°Fahrenehit for 18-minutes. Toss twice during cook time. Season with salt, pepper, and other seasonings.

Nutritional Values per serving: Calories: 42, Total Fat: 1.3g, Carbs: 2.1g, Protein: 1.4g

Spicy Mango Okra

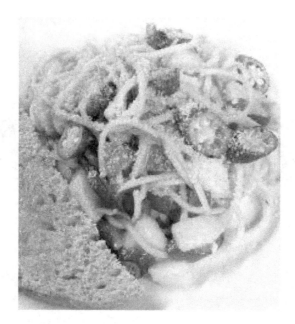

Cook Time: 25 minutes

Servings: 5

Ingredients:

35-ounces Okra, washed, drained and wiped dry

1 teaspoon red chili powder

2 tablespoons coriander powder

2 tablespoons almond flour

1 ½ tablespoons olive oil

Pinch of caraway seeds

Pinch of Fenugreek seeds

Pinch of Asafoetida

½ teaspoon turmeric

2 green chilies

4 teaspoons dry mango powder

Salt to taste

Directions:

Slit the okra lengthwise into half. Brush some olive oil on okra then fry in the air fryer. Heat some oil in a pan and add the asafetida, heating it for 10-seconds.   Add the fenugreek and caraway seeds, fry them for 10-seconds. Stir in the almond flour and cook for 10-minutes. Mix in the air fried okra and sprinkle the spices on top. Cook for 10-minutes, adding the green chilies cook for an additional 2-minutes.

Nutritional Values per serving: Calories: 35, Total Fat: 0.11g, Carbs: 7.7g, Protein: 2.27g

Honey Roasted Carrots

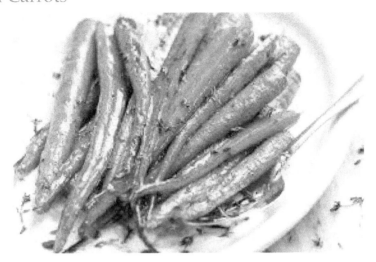

Cook Time: 25 minutes

Servings: 4

Ingredients:

3 cups baby carrots

1 tablespoon olive oil

1 tablespoon honey

Salt and pepper to taste

Directions:

Toss all the ingredients in a bowl. Cook for 12-minutes in an air fryer at 390°Fahrenheit.

Nutritional Values per serving: Calories: 82, Total Fat: 3.2g, Carbs: 2.1g, Protein: 1.0g

Hot Pepper Pin Wheel

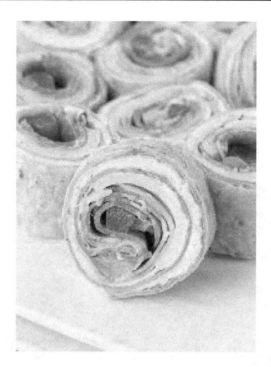

Cook Time: 6 minutes

Servings: 3

Ingredients:

2 lbs. dill pickles

3 almond tortillas

Salt and pepper to taste

3-ounces sliced ham

1 lb. softened cream

1 hot pepper, finely diced

Directions:

Mix diced hot pepper in with cheese. On one side of the tortilla spread cheese over it. Place the ham slice over it. Spread a layer of cheese on top of ham slice. Roll 1 pickle up in the tortilla. Preheat the air fryer to 340°Fahrenheit. Place the rolls in air fryer basket and cook for 6-minutes.

Nutritional Values per serving: Calories: 67, Total Fat: 2.1g, Carbs: 0.11g, Protein: 3.2g

Lemon Courgette Caviar

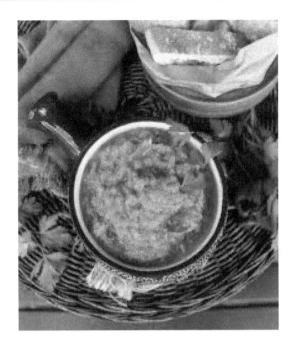

Cook Time: 20 minutes

Servings: 3

Ingredients:

2 medium Courgettes

1 tablespoon olive oil

1 ½ tablespoons balsamic vinegar

½ red onion

Juice of one lemon

Directions:

Preheat your air fryer. Wash, then dry courgettes. Add lemon juice to over courgettes. Arrange courgettes in a baking dish, then bake them in the air fryer for 20-minutes. Remove the courgettes from the oven and allow them to cool. Blend the onion in a blender. Slice the courgettes in half, lengthwise, then remove their insides using a spoon. Place courgettes into mixer and process everything. Add the vinegar, the olive oil and a little bit of salt, then blend again. Serve cool with tomato sauce.

Nutritional Values per serving: Calories: 76, Total Fat: 0.3g, Carbs: 18g, Protein: 3g

Parmesan Asparagus Fries

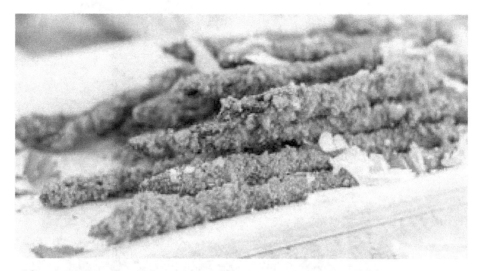

Cook Time: 10 minutes

Servings: 5

Ingredients:

1 lb. asparagus spears

¼ cup almond flour

Salt and pepper to taste

2 eggs, beaten

½ cup Parmesan cheese, grated

1 cup pork rinds

Directions:

Preheat your air fryer to 380°Fahrenheit. Combine pork rinds and parmesan cheese in a small bowl. Season with salt and pepper. Line baking sheet with parchment paper. First, dip half the asparagus spears into flour, then into eggs, and finally into pork rind mixture. Place asparagus spears on the baking sheet and bake for 10-minutes. Repeat with remaining spears.

Nutritional Values per serving: Calories: 20, Total Fat: 0.1g, Carbs: 3.9g, Protein: 2.2g

Garlic & Parsley Roasted Mushrooms

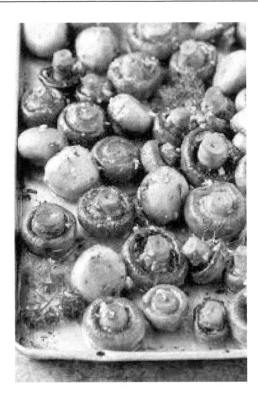

Cook Time: 30 minutes

Servings: 4

Ingredients:

2 lbs. mushrooms, washed, quartered, dried

1 tablespoon duck fat

½ teaspoon garlic powder

2 teaspoons Herbes de Provence

2 tablespoons white vermouth

1 teaspoon parsley, fresh, finely chopped

Directions:

Place the duck fat, garlic powder, Herbes de Provence in an air fryer pan and heat for 2-minutes. Stir in the mushrooms. Cook for 25-minutes at 300°Fahrenheit. Mix in the vermouth and cook for an additional 5-minutes. Sprinkle mushrooms with parsley for garnish.

Nutritional Values per serving: Calories: 92, Total Fat: 0.23g, Carbs: 0.52g, Protein: 1.2g

Grilled Pineapple with Cinnamon

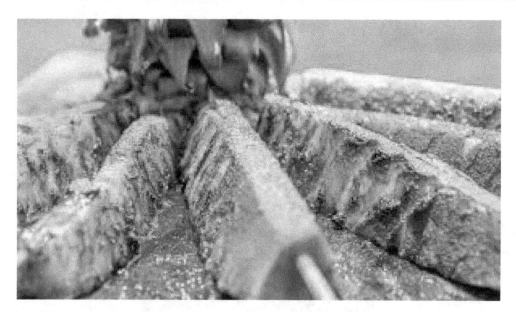

Cook Time: 20 minutes

Servings: 2

Ingredients:

4 pineapple slices

2 tablespoons Truvia

1 teaspoon cinnamon

Directions:

Add the cinnamon and Truvia into a Ziploc bag and shake well. Add the pineapple slices to it and shake and coat. Leave to marinate in the fridge for 20-minutes. Preheat your air fryer for 5-minutes at 360°Fahrenheit. Place the pineapple pieces on the air fryer rack and grill them for 10-minutes. Flip and grill them for an additional 10-minutes.

Nutritional Values per serving: Calories: 276, Total Fat: 5.3g, Carbs: 4.2g, Protein: 4.6g

Ginger & Honey Cauliflower Bites

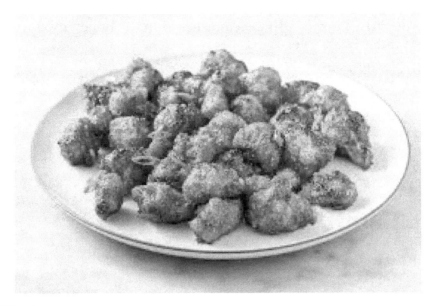

Cook Time: 20 minutes

Servings: 4

Ingredients:

1 head of cauliflower, cut into florets

1/3 cup oats

1/3 cup almond flour

1 egg, beaten

1 teaspoon mixed spice

2 tablespoons soy sauce

2 tablespoons honey

Salt and pepper to taste

½ teaspoon mustard powder

1 teaspoon mixed herbs

1/3 cup desiccated coconut

1 teaspoon ginger powder

Directions:

Preheat your air fryer to 360°Fahrenheit. In a bowl, combine flour, oats, ginger powder and coconut. Season it with salt and pepper. Add egg into another bowl. Season the cauliflower florets with the mixed herbs, salt, and pepper. Dip florets into the egg and then dredge in coconut mix. Cook in your air fryer for 15-minutes at 315°Fahrenheit. Mix remaining ingredients in a bowl. Dip the cauliflower in the honey mixture and cook for an additional 5-minutes in air fryer.

Nutritional Values per serving: Calories: 42, Total Fat: 2.3g, Carbs: 3.1g, Protein: 3.2g

Baked Tomato & Egg

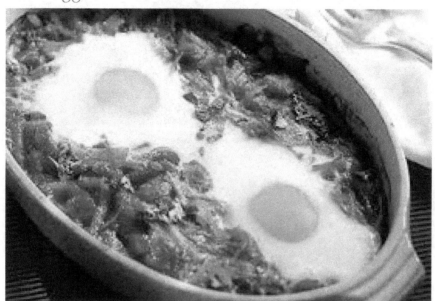

Cook Time: 20 minutes

Servings: 2

Ingredients:

2 tomatoes

4 eggs

1 cup mozzarella cheese, shredded

Salt and pepper to taste

1 tablespoon olive oil

A few basil leaves

Directions:

Preheat your air fryer to 360°Fahrenheit. Cut each tomato into two halves and place them in a bowl. Season with salt and pepper. Place cheese around the bottom of the tomatoes and add the basil leaves. Break one egg into each tomato slice. Garnish with cheese and drizzle with olive oil. Set the temperature to 360°Fahrenheit and bake for 20-minutes.

Nutritional Values per serving: Calories: 28.9, Total Fat: 2.4g, Carbs: 2.0g, Protein: 0.4g

Paprika Chips

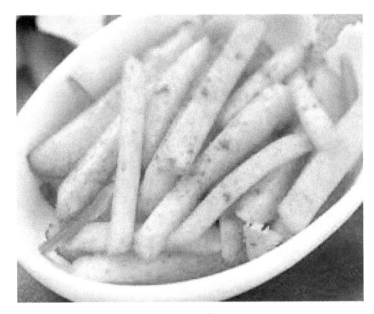

Cook Time: 40 minutes

Servings: 4

Ingredients:

31-ounces of sweet potatoes, peeled and cut into chips

½ teaspoon salt

2 tablespoons olive oil

½ tablespoon paprika

Directions:

Toss all the ingredients together in a bowl. Place in a pan inside your air fryer and cook for 40-minutes at 300°Fahrenheit.

Nutritional Values per serving: Calories: 62, Total Fat: 6.5g, Carbs: 41.5g, Protein: 5.3g

French Beans with Walnuts & Almonds

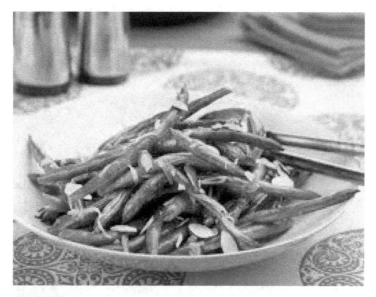

Cook Time: 27 minutes

Servings: 6

Ingredients:

1 ½ lbs. of French green beans

 (stems removed)

¼ cup slivered almonds (lightly toasted)

¼ cup walnuts, finely chopped

½ teaspoon ground white pepper

½ lb. shallots, peeled and quartered

1 teaspoon sea salt

2 tablespoons olive oil

Directions:

Boil some water in a pan, adding the green beans to it. Cook beans for 2-minutes with salt. Drain the beans. Place the green beans into a bowl and toss with the rest of the ingredients except the walnuts and almonds. Mix nuts together in small bowl and set aside. Place into air fryer basket and cook for 25-minutes at 400°Fahrenheit. Toss twice during cook time. Serve garnished with mixed nuts.

Nutritional Values per serving: Calories: 213, Total Fat: 5.2g, Carbs: 3.4g, Protein: 4.3g

Crab & Cheese Soufflé

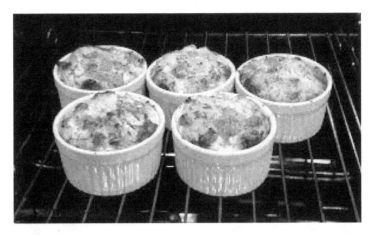

Cook Time: 18 minutes

Servings: 2

Ingredients:

1 lb. cooked crab meat

1 capsicum

1 small onion, diced

1 cup cream

1 cup milk

4-ounces Brie

Brandy to cover crab meat

3 eggs

5 drops liquid stevia

3-ounces cheddar cheese, grated

4 cups bread, cubed

Directions:

Soak the cram meat in brandy and 4-parts water. Loosen the meat in brandy. Sautė onion and bread. Grate cheddar cheese and mix ingredients. In the same pan, add some of the butter and stir for a minute. Add the crab to pan. Add ½ of the milk and 1 tablespoon of brandy and cook for 2-minutes. Add the bread cubes to frying pan and mix well. Sprinkle with cheese and pepper. Put the stuffing in 5 ramekins, without brushing them with oil. Distribute the brie evenly. In a bowl, combine ½ cup of cream with stevia. Heat the cream in a pan and add remaining milk. Pour mixture into ramekins. Preheat your air fryer to 350°Fahreneheit add dish and cook for 20-minutes.

Broccoli with Cheese & Olives

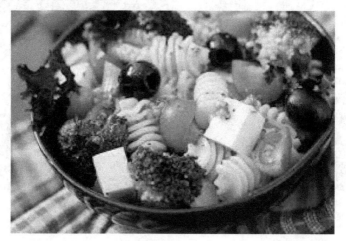

Cook Time: 15 minutes

Servings: 4

Ingredients:

2lbs. broccoli florets

¼ cup parmesan cheese, shaved

2 teaspoons lemon zest, grated

1/3 cup Kalamata olives, halved, pitted

½ teaspoon ground black pepper

1 teaspoon sea salt

2 tablespoons olive oil

Directions:

Boil the water in a pan and cook the broccoli for 4-minutes. Drain broccoli. Toss the broccoli with oil, salt, and pepper. Place broccoli in your air fryer basket and cook for 15-minutes at 400°Fahrenheit. Toss twice during cook time. Move to a serving bowl and toss in lemon zest, olives, and cheese.

Nutritional Values per serving: Calories: 242, Total Fat: 7.2g, Carbs: 3.2g, Protein: 5.6g

Spicy Mozzarella Stick

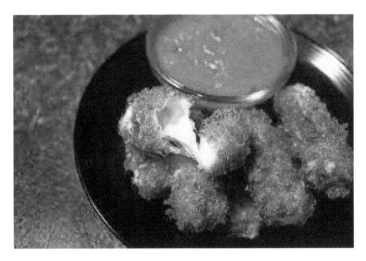

Cook Time: 5 minutes

Servings: 3

Ingredients:

8-ounces mozzarella cheese, cut into strips

2 tablespoons olive oil

½ teaspoon salt

1 cup pork rinds

1 egg

1 teaspoon garlic powder

1 teaspoon paprika

Directions:

Cut the mozzarella into 6 strips. Whisk the egg along with salt, paprika, and garlic powder. Dip the mozzarella strips into egg mixture first, then into pork rinds. Arrange them on a baking platter and place in the fridge for 30-minutes. Preheat your air fryer to 360°Fahrenheit. Drizzle olive oil into the air fryer. Arrange the mozzarella sticks in the air fryer and cook for about 5-minutes. Make sure to turn them at least twice, to ensure they will become golden on all sides.

Nutritional Values per serving: Calories: 156, Total Fat: 9.6g, Carbs: 1.89g, Protein: 16g

Fried Zucchini, Squash, & Carrot Mix

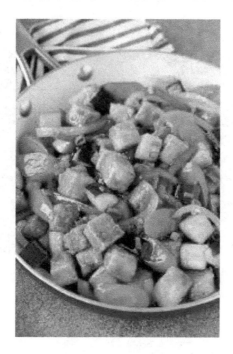

Cook Time: 35 minutes

Servings: 4

Ingredients:

½ lb. carrots, peeled and cubed

6 teaspoons olive oil

1 lb. zucchini, chopped into half-moons

1 lb. yellow squash, chopped in half-moons

1 teaspoon sea salt

½ teaspoon white pepper

1 tablespoon Tarragon leaves, chopped

Directions:

Toss carrots in a bowl with 2 teaspoons of olive oil, then place them into air fryer basket. Cook for 5-minutes at 400°Fahrenheit. Toss the zucchini and squash in the rest of the oil, salt and pepper and place into air fryer. Cook for 30-minutes, tossing three times during cook time. Toss with tarragon and serve.

Nutritional Values per serving: Calories: 217, Total Fat: 4.2g, Carbs: 3.9g, Protein: 6.2g

Parsley & Garlic Flavored Potatoes

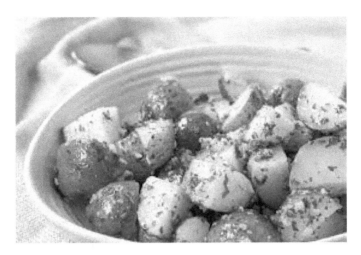

Cook Time: 40 minutes

Servings: 4

Ingredients:

3 Idaho baking potatoes (pricked with a fork)

2 tablespoons olive oil

1 teaspoon parsley

1 tablespoon garlic, minced

Salt to taste

Directions:

Stir ingredients together in a bowl. Rub the potatoes with the mix. Place them into air fryer basket and cook for 40-minutes at 390°Fahrenheit. Toss twice during cook time.

Nutritional Values per serving: Calories: 97, Total Fat: 0.64g, Carbs: 25.2g, Protein: 10.2g

Hot Spicy Thyme Cherry Tomatoes

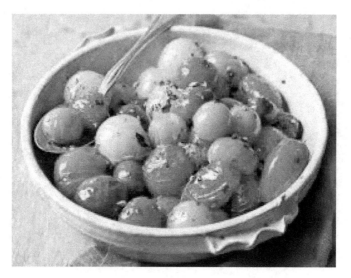

Cook Time: 25 minutes

Servings: 4

Ingredients:

1 dozen cherry tomatoes

1 tablespoon olive oil

½ teaspoon thyme, dried

Salt and pepper to taste

1 garlic clove, minced

1 teaspoon paprika

Directions:

Chop the tomatoes in half and discard the seeds. Toss the tomatoes with the rest of the ingredients in a bowl. Place in the air fryer at 390°Fahrenheit for 15-minutes.

Nutritional Values per serving: Calories: 232, Total Fat: 5.2g, Carbs: 4.3g, Protein: 5.1g

Conclusion

I hope that your air fryer is giving you lots of joy, time and most importantly, tasty dishes. Please feel free to adjust and alter these recipes, or simply use them as a springboard of inspiration for your own creations!

Putting together interesting and unexpected ingredients is so much fun and can be really rewarding, so get creative in your kitchen.

Always remember to clean your air fryer and accessories according to the instructions and safety precautions after each cooking adventure.

Like every appliance, maintenance is needed to get what you would like in the device. Any tool employed for preparing food must be stored spotlessly clean. Don't let dirt develop and clean the environment fryer frequently so you get great results any time you make use of the air fryer. You have to make certain you retain it keep clean and maintain it for results efficiently along with a taken care of appliance always lasts longer. We provides you with some cleanings tips, however it is not difficult. The outdoors and inside parts could be cleaned fairly easily and ought to be done frequently. Within the situation from the heating coil, get it done a couple of occasions annually only.

Bariatric Air Fryer Cookbook

70+ Healthy, Tasty Recipes for After-Surgery Recovery and Lifelong Weight Management

By

Chef Mirco Miccio

Table of Contents

Introduction

Weight loss surgery has proved to be an invaluable tool in the process of losing weight and becoming healthier. However, this tool must be used correctly in order to achieve positive results. The most important step is to follow your doctor's Directions and accordingly try to ease back into eating and taking care of your healing body. In the long-term, you must be careful of not only your portion sizes and also of what foods are good for you and which ones you should avoid.

Bariatric surgery, on its own, is not enough to enable you to lose weight and keep it off. After the bariatric surgery, your diet will have to change drastically. You will need to follow a healthy diet of bariatric recipes to ensure your long-term weight loss.

Eat healthy

The most important step in following a bariatric diet is to eat healthily.

. In general, your bariatric diet should consist only of 'FOG' foods, which are as follows:

Farm- The food that is raised on farms i.e. chicken, eggs, dairy products.

Ocean- The food that comes from the ocean i.e. fish.

Ground- The food that is grown in the ground i.e. fruits, vegetables, nuts, whole grains.

Proteins-the essential part of diet

Proteins are one of the most important nutrients required by your body. You need up to 80 grams/day of proteins, in order to stay healthy. However, now that your stomach is down to the size of a golf ball, 80 grams is a big percentage of the available space.

If you are not eating enough proteins, your body will begin to break down muscle, in order to get the number of proteins required by the body.

This can cause nausea, irritability, weakness, and tiredness.

Proteins can be found in a number of foods including, meat, fish, dairy products, legumes, and nuts.

Stages of a bariatric diet

The stages of a bariatric diet in the first few months may vary, depending on the type of weight loss surgery you had. This is a general, four-stage plan for successful healing and weight loss process. However, it is important to follow your surgeon and dietitian's Directions, before you follow any diet.

Stage 1: clear liquids

Basically, clear liquids, as the name implies, are liquids you can see through. Apart from water, there are several other liquids, which are included in this category as well:

- Pulp-free juices that have been diluted 50/50 with water (however, orange juice and tomato juice are not considered clear liquids)

- Clear beef, chicken, or vegetable broth (high-protein broths)

- Clear, sugar-free gelatin

- Sugar-free ice pops

- Decaf coffee

- tea

- Sugar-free, noncarbonated fruit drinks

- Flavored sugar-free, noncarbonated water

- Clear liquid supplements

Stage 2: full liquids

Full liquids are liquids or semi-liquids, which are pourable at room temperature. You also cannot see through them. You can start to have these liquids as early as the second day after surgery, provided you can tolerate clear liquids.

Full liquids include all those liquids which are in their clear liquid phase as well as the following foods:

- Low-fat soups that have been strained or puréed.

- Cooked wheat or rice cereals that have been thinned and are of a soupy consistency

- All juices (diluted fruit juice, 50/50 with water)

- Skimmed or 1 percent milk; plain, low-fat soy milk; or buttermilk (or lactose-free milk if you're lactose intolerant)

- Sugar-free custards or puddings

- Sugar-free hot chocolate

- Protein shakes with at least 10 grams of protein per 100 calories

- No-sugar-added or light yogurt

Stage 3: smooth foods

Smooth foods, also known as puréed foods, are those foods which have been put through the food processor in order to turn them into a puree with a smooth texture. You may follow the stage three for up to four weeks, depending on your surgeon's recommendations.

Smooth foods include the following:

- Blended low-fat cottage cheese

- Blended scrambled eggs

- Mashed potatoes made with skim milk

- Sugar-free applesauce

- Blended meats

- Part-skim ricotta cheese

Stage 4: soft foods

The stage 4 diet is the easiest to follow, as you can easily fulfill your protein requirements without using supplements. Your diet can include the following soft foods:

- Finely ground tuna

- Soft, tender, moist proteins like chicken salad (no onions or celery), turkey, veal, pork, beef, shrimp, scallops, and white fish that have been minced or ground in the food processor

- Soft, cooked vegetables

- Canned fruit packed in its own juice or water

- Eggs

- Low-fat soft cheese

- Low-fat cottage cheese

- Beans

- Crackers

Bariatric recipes

A good bariatric recipe is one which is high in protein and low in fat. Fish and lean meat are the excellent sources of proteins. Fried foods and recipes with lots of oil and butter must be avoided at all costs. Therefore, baking and grilling is a better option than frying. Spices and lemon juice can also be used, as they provide healthier flavors as compared to the oil and butter.

You should also try to avoid foods that are heavy in carbohydrates like pasta or white bread. Whole wheat bread and brown rice are better alternatives.

Best ways to prepare bariatric recipes

The preparation of bariatric food is the most important step in determining whether the food is healthy and meets all the requirements of a bariatric diet. Therefore, the following things must be kept in mind, when preparing your food:

- The food must be baked, grilled, poached or broiled. Frying is not an option.

- Use skimmed milk instead of whole milk.

- Use chicken or vegetable broth instead of oil.

- Oil must be replaced with applesauce or yogurt.

- Add spices or lemon juice to add flavors instead of olive oil or butter.

Chapter 1: Tips for Weight Loss

This is by no means an exhaustive list but just something to let you kick start the weight loss journey if you haven't already. The tips are all quickly actionable and easy to follow, though some may require a little more effort than the other, these are all ideas which have been known to work for people in pursuit of weight loss.

Record what you eat – Get a notebook if you are of the more pen and paper variety, or simply just use the note function on your smartphone to record down the food that you are consuming throughout the day. This gives you a sense of accountability when you sit down at the end of the day and review what you have eaten. You might be surprised at the amount of food you have taken in, and this will serve as a timely reminder to do better the next day. Get an accountability partner – Many people do better in tasks that require discipline when they are required to report to somebody else.

Getting an accountability partner will give that added sense of responsibility as well as the desire not to disappoint the partner when you report on your weight loss daily activities. Having someone to cajole and encourage you during this period can also be immensely gratifying, and that could be the added push to keep you on track for the weight loss journey.

Get enough sleep – It is by no means a measure of surprise to know that lack of sleep hampers your weight loss efforts by the simple increase of the hormone cortisol in our body system. Cortisol increases our appetite and hunger sensations, which is why getting sufficient sleep can do simple wonders in letting you shed the excess pounds. You will feel less cranky and more energized too!

Be mindful when eating – We get the feeling of fullness and satiation when we concentrate on the food that we are chewing and not get distracted by the ever-present mobile devices or the other assorted distractions available in this modern world while we have our meals. When eating, just eat! I know, it is easier said than done, but you can try counting the number of chews for that mouthful of food, get to seven or ten chews before swallowing. It helps to focus your mind back onto the food that you consume, and as a bonus, you are helping your stomach with better digestion as well!

Avoid processed foods – Yeap, that means the ice-creams, donuts and creamy cakes have got to take a backseat when it comes to your food selection. Pile on the whole and natural foods because those are nutrient dense items that will ensure you do not take in empty calories. Most of the processed food found today contain quite a bit of sugar and are pretty much deficient in the nutrients department, hence the term empty calories! The sugar eats into your daily calorie limit while not providing you with the essential nutrients your body needs. Go for chicken meat instead of chicken nuggets, whole potatoes instead of fries. You get the idea. Putting whole foods on your platter gives you more bang for the buck regarding your daily calorie limit, where you ensure that the calories you take in supplies your body with the nutrients that it needs to function well.

How can Hypnosis change the way you think?

Human information on the genuine substance of daze and entrancing is gotten from the Assumption Satisfaction Hypothesis of Dreams by Joe Griffin. For, obviously, dreaming is the most profound daze of all. At the point when the baby initially starts to show REM (quick eye development) rest, it is the most crucial type of daze that creates in the belly. Dreams deactivate the enthusiastic excitement, permitting the mind to react newly to each new day, thus safeguarding our senses' uprightness.

Because of the reasonable physiological similitudes with the territory of REM rest, we allude to daze as the REM state in the human giving methodology.

Profound daze reflects numerous parts of REM rest when instigated by spellbinding, for example, impenetrability to outside tangible data, less agony affectability, muscle loss of motion, and so forth Moreover, parts of how the REM state functions when we dream equal techniques utilized for daze enlistment. To help create daze, numerous hypnotists may utilize cadenced movement (for instance, making dull hand developments or getting people to gaze at turning optical figments), which connections back to the crude cerebrum of fish that we have advanced from. Obviously, on account of their consistent need to move, steer and equilibrium themselves in water, which they do by 'turning' their balances, fish respond incredibly capably to cadence. Centering consideration mirrors retention in a fantasy. Another closeness is in the focal point of consideration: creating a noisy clamor or unexpected development can place an individual in a daze, as that quickly catches their consideration and includes electrical cerebrum action known as the direction reaction, a similar PGO waves as found in REM rest. The direction reaction fires angrily when we initially begin to dream.

The fantasy hypothesis of assumption satisfaction clarifies that this is the instrument for making the mind aware of the presence of unexpressed passionate feelings of excitement that should be released in a fantasy. Considerably more likenesses exist. As we nod off, the profound unwinding that psychotherapists use as enlistment into daze matches what occurs. Also, whenever clients are loose, the guided symbolism we use to permit them to see and beat their issues from an alternate point of view equal dream material emerging, the distinction being that the advisor manages the interaction in a misleadingly incited daze, while the 'fantasy script symbolism' in our rest gives the 'unused enthusiastic feelings of excitement from the earlier day.' As we probably are aware, allegory, when given to an individual in a daze, is profoundly incredible in treatment; and dreams are illustrations. Clear daze encounters may include mental trips. For instance, clients may report the glow of the sun they envisioned on their appearances, and dreams are additionally illusory. Exploration has shown that in the two conditions, a similar cerebrum pathways are dynamic. Likewise, visionaries additionally immediately experience wonders that can be actuated in a daze, like an amnesia (for the fantasy), sedation and absense of pain, body hallucinations, catalepsy, separation, and twisting of time.

Be that as it may, similarly as spellbinding isn't a daze, so the REM state isn't a fantasy. In actuality, it is the venue wherein the fantasy happens. The fantasy script isn't like the REM theater, our inward 'reality generator' as Joe Griffin appeared, and inside, it is carried on or made genuine.

In a wide range of daze, the REM state at that point is dynamic. It's not simply a condition of 'loose' or 'latent.' It's dynamic. All types of learning, scholarly or something else (counting molding, treatment, and teaching), are engaged with programming inborn and learned information, and furthermore when we wander off in fantasy land and take care of issues. At the point when we are damaged, the REM state is the medium through which the mind catches the horrible mishap and turns into a learned part of the models of endurance. Along these lines, the REM state, especially on the off chance that we are associated with conveying treatment, is fundamentally critical to comprehend.

Chapter 2: Breakfast

Italian Poached Eggs

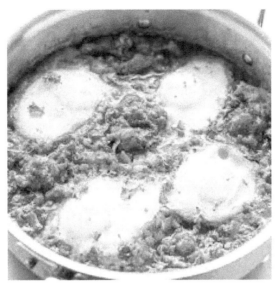

Serves: 6

Time: 30 minutes

Ingredients

16 oz. marinara sauce

4 shredded basil leaves

3-4 roasted red pepper, sliced

Pepper

4 eggs

Salt

Directions

Grab a skillet and let it heat up. Add the marinara sauce and the peppers then mix them together and allow them to heat up.

Once they are hot, use a spoon to make four wells into the marinara sauce. Now, crack one egg into each of the wells you have made.

Sprinkle pepper and salt over each of the eggs.

Allow this to cook for about 12 minutes. You can cook the eggs as long as you want until it reaches your desired doneness. You can also place a lid on your skillet so that the eggs cook a bit faster.

Remove the skillet from the stove and sprinkle the torn basil over the top. Scoop the eggs out along with a bit of sauce and enjoy.

Egg Burrito

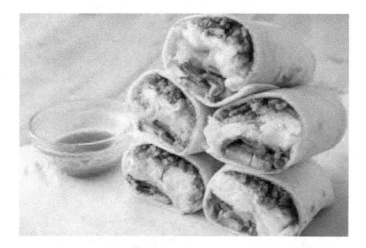

Serves: 4

Time: 30 minutes

Ingredients

Pepper

1 tbsp. shredded Mexican cheese blend

Salt

2 tbsp. salsa

1 egg + 1 egg white

1 oz. protein of choices such as ground beef, chicken, or tofu

2 tbsp. plain fat-free Greek yogurt

Directions

Place the egg white and egg into a small bowl. Whisk until well combined. Spray cooking spray on a skillet. When warmed, pour eggs into the hot pan. Tilt pan to spread the eggs evenly on the bottom. Let it sit until edges are set. Sprinkle with pepper and salt then gently flip over.

Allow the other side to cook until the eggs are done. Place on a plate. Put your protein of choice and cheese onto the center of the egg. Roll up the egg in the form of a burrito. Add salsa and Greek yogurt, if desired.

Bunless Breakfast Sandwich

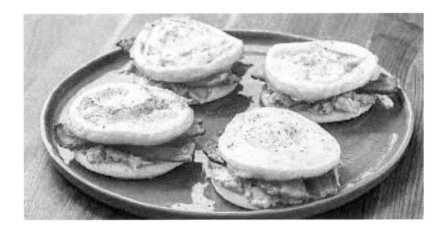

Serves: 4

Time: 35 minutes

Ingredients

¼ c shredded cheddar cheese

2 eggs

2 tbsp. water

½ avocado, mashed

2 sliced cooked bacon

Directions

Place two canning jar lids into a skillet and spray with cooking spray. Let everything warm up. Crack one egg in each lid and whisk the egg gently with a fork to break the yolks.

Pour a small amount of water into the pan and put the lid on the skillet. Allow to cook and steam the eggs. Cook for three minutes. Take off the lid and put cheese on just one of the eggs. Allow cheese to melt for about one minute.

Put the egg without the cheese on a plate. Add avocado and then the bacon on top. Put the other egg on top with the cheesy side down. Enjoy.

Chocolate Porridge

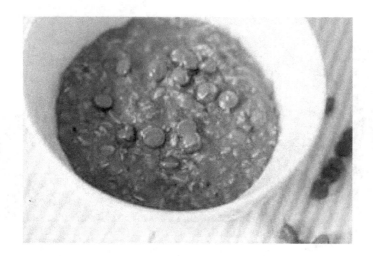

Serves: 4

Time: 5 minutes

Ingredients

Chopped nuts, fruits, or seeds of choice

4 tbsp. porridge oats

1 c skim milk

Sugar-free syrup

1 square dark unsweetened chocolate

1 tbsp. cocoa powder

Directions

Place the chocolate, cocoa powder, oats, and milk in a microwavable bowl.

Cook for two minutes. Give everything a good stir and cook for an additional 15 to 20 seconds.

Put in a serving bowl and add desired toppings. Enjoy.

Cheesy Spiced Pancakes

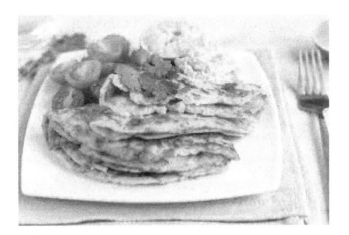

Serves: 4

Time: 55 minutes

Ingredients

Pancakes:

1 tbsp. artificial sweetener

1 tsp. mixed spice, ground

Low-fat cooking spray

8 oz. spreadable goat cheese

Pinch salt

3 eggs, separated

½ c all-purpose flour

Optional Adult Toppings:

Sweetener

1 measure Brandy

4 tangerines, peeled

2 oz. cranberries

Directions

To make the pancakes: Combine the egg yolks, cheese, and mixed spice. Add the salt and flour and mix well.

Beat the egg whites until they are stiff peaks and whisk in sweetener. Fold this into the cheese mixture.

If using the optional topping, place sweetener and tangerines into a pot. Stir occasionally until tangerines begin to release some juices and begin to look a bit syrupy. Add the Brandy and cranberries. Let this cook for few minutes. Keep warm until ready to use.

Spray the skillet with cooking spray. Allow to warm up. Add three large spoonful of batter into the pan. Cook for about two minutes until bubbles form on top. Flip and cook until the other side is browned. Remove from the pan and keep warm. Continue until all batter has been used. You should get 12 pancakes from this batter.

Divide among four plates and spoon the topping. Enjoy.

Pumpkin Pie Oatmeal

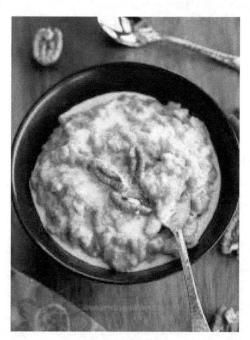

Serves: 6

Time: 10 minutes

Ingredients

½ c canned pumpkin

1 tsp. Truvia

Dash ground cloves

1/3 c old fashioned oats

Dash ground ginger

½ c no salt 1% cottage cheese

1/8 tsp. cinnamon

Directions

Place the sweetener, spices, pumpkin, and oats into a microwavable bowl. Mix to combine. Microwave on high for 90 seconds. Add the cottage cheese and stir well. Microwave for another 60 seconds. Wait for few minutes before eating then enjoy.

Egg Muffin

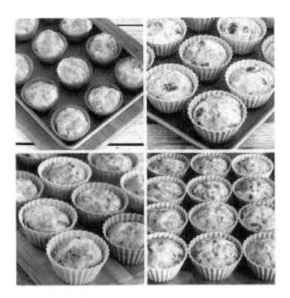

Serves: 4

Time: 45 minutes

Ingredients

¼ tsp. salt

12 slices turkey bacon

¼ tsp. Italian seasoning

6 large eggs

¼ tsp. pepper

¾ c shredded low-fat shredded cheese of choice

½ c 1% milk

Directions

Spray cooking spray into muffin pan. Your oven needs to be warmed to 350.

Place three slices of bacon on the bottom of each muffin cup.

Mix all remaining ingredients together until well combined. Reserve ¼ cup of shredded cheese. Put a fourth cup of this mixture into every muffin cup. Add a bit more cheese on top.

Bake for about 25 minutes. The eggs should be set.

Flour-Less Pancakes

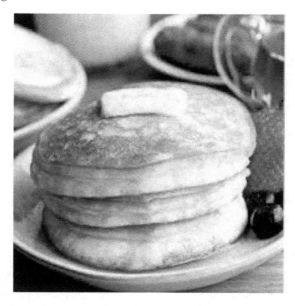

Serves: 8

Time: 70 minutes

Ingredients

Milk to mix

1 egg

Low-fat cooking spray

1 c rolled oats

1 banana

Directions

Place the banana, egg, and oats into a food processor. Process until smooth. Add a small amount of milk and blend again. Add the milk until the mixture has reached a runny consistency. Three tablespoons should be the maximum amount you use.

Allow to sit for about 15 minutes. This lets the mixture thicken slightly.

Spray a small amount of cooking spray into a skillet. Allow to get warm. Add a spoonful of the batter to form a small pancake. Put as many as your pan will allow. Just make sure you have room to flip each. Allow the first side to cook for about a minute until bubbles begin to form on the surface. Flip and cook until browned. Remove from the skillet onto a plate and keep warm while you continue to cook the remaining batter.

Serve warm with fruit, yogurt, sugar-free syrup, a dusting of powdered sugar, or a drizzle of lemon. You might prefer them plain. Either way, enjoy.

Broccoli Quiche

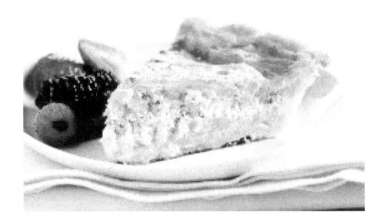

Serves: 4

Time: 60 minutes

Ingredients

½ c fat-free half and half

3 oz. low-fat Swiss cheese

¼ c skim milk

½ c canned mushrooms

1 c egg substitute

1 large head broccoli

Directions

Your oven should be set to 400. Coat a pie plate with nonstick spray.

Put the broccoli in a steamer basket. In a pot that the basket will fit into, add about an inch of water. Place a steamer basket into the pot then steam for about five minutes. Allow to cool slightly then give the broccoli a rough chop.

Put the mushrooms and broccoli into the pie plate.

Whisk together the half and half, skim milk, and egg substitute. Whisk until well combined.

Pour the egg mixture over the mushrooms and broccoli. Add some cheese on top.

Cook for about 40 minutes until the eggs are set.

Cut into four equal servings and enjoy.

Oatmeal Cookie Shake

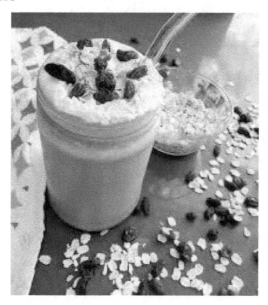

Serves: 8

Time: 20 minutes

Ingredients

Low-fat cream, cinnamon, and nuts – garnish

1 c low-fat nut milk

Ice

½ tsp. cinnamon

¼ tsp. vanilla

1 scoop vanilla whey protein powder

1 tbsp. oatmeal

Directions

Place the protein powder, mice, milk, vanilla, cinnamon, and oatmeal into a strong blender, and pulse couple of times until all of the ingredients come together.

Pour the shake into a glass and top with some cinnamon, cream, and nuts.

Soft Eggs with Chives and Ricotta

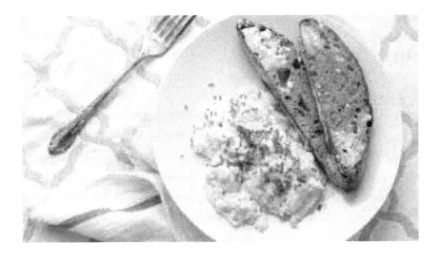

Serves: 4

Time: 40 minutes

Ingredients

2 eggs

Olive oil

½ c milk

1 tbsp. chopped chives

½ c ricotta

Directions

Add the eggs and milk to a jar. Place the lid on tightly and shake it until everything is mixed together well.

Grab yourself a skillet and place it on the stove. Once it is warm, pour the eggs into the skillet and scramble them. Allow them to cook until they are soft-set. Once soft-set, let it cook and gently stir them once in a while.

After the eggs are done, stir the ricotta and the chives. Add the eggs to a plate and drizzle some oil over the top if you would like.

Ham and Egg Roll-Ups

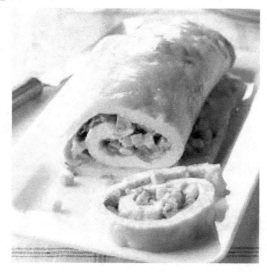

Serves: 6

Time: 35 minutes

Ingredients

2 tsp. garlic powder

1 c baby spinach

1 c chopped tomatoes

10 eggs

Pepper

2 tbsp. butter

Salt

1 ½ c shredded cheddar cheese

20 ham slices

Directions

Turn oven to broil. Crack all the eggs into a bowl and beat together. Add the garlic powder, pepper, and salt. Mix well.

Warm a skillet on stove top. Add the butter and allow it to melt. Add the eggs and scramble until they are done. Mix the cheese, stirring until it melts. Fold in the spinach and tomatoes.

Put two pieces of ham on a cutting board. Add a spoonful of eggs then roll up. Repeat this process until all ham and eggs are used.

Place the roll-ups on a baking sheet and broil about five minutes.

Cottage Cheese Pancakes

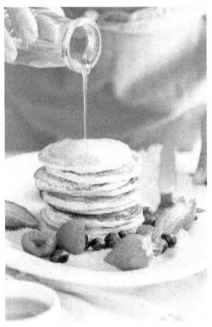

Serves: 7

Time: 45 minutes

Ingredients

1/3 c all-purpose flour

½ tbsp. canola oil

½ tsp. baking soda

3 eggs, lightly beaten

1 c low-fat cottage cheese

Directions

Sift the baking soda and flour in a small bowl.

Mix the remaining ingredients together.

Mix the flour into the wet ingredients and stir to incorporate.

Spray cooking spray into a skillet and warm. When warmed, place one-third cup of the batter into the pan and cook until you see bubbles. Flip and cook until the other side is browned.

Serve warm with sugar-free syrup. Enjoy.

Mocha Frappuccino

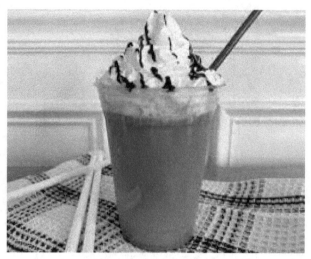

Serves: 4

Time: 15 minutes

Ingredients

¼ c brewed coffee

Low-sugar chocolate syrup

¼ c unsweetened almond milk

Low-fat whipped cream

½ c 0% fat Greek yogurt

1 c ice

3-4 drops liquid sweetener

1 tbsp. cocoa powder

Directions

Place the coffee, ice, milk, cocoa, yogurt, and sweetener in a blender and pulse until all of the ingredients come together and it's all smooth.

Pour the Frappuccino into a glass and swirl some whipped cream and chocolate syrup over the top.

PB&J Pancakes

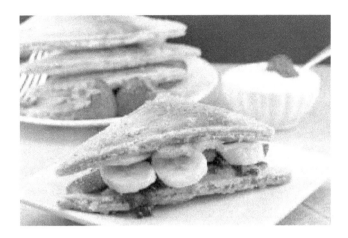

Serves: 8

Time: 50 minutes

Ingredients

½ c instant oatmeal

1 c frozen mixed berries

½ c low-fat cottage cheese

4 large egg whites

2 tbsp. powdered peanuts

Directions

The ingredients have to be put in the blender in a specific order. You will add the cottage cheese first. Next, will be the oatmeal. Followed by the powdered peanuts. Last, will be the egg whites. Blend until smooth and the consistency is of a pancake batter. Pour into a bowl and add the mixed fruit. Spray a skillet with cooking spray. Put ¼ cup batter into the heated skillet and cook until the top forms bubbles. Flip and cook until browned on the other side. Should make between four and seven pancakes. Serve warm with sugar-free syrup.

Breakfast Popsicles

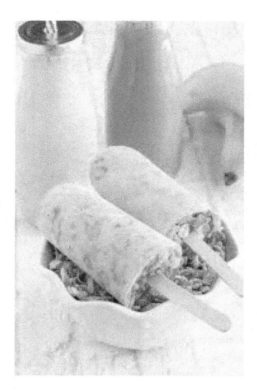

Serves: 4

Time: 50 minutes

Ingredients

½ c oats

1 c Greek yogurt

1 c mixed berries

½ c 1% milk

Directions

Mix together the yogurt and milk. Divide the mixture equally into popsicle molds. Place some berries into each one. Divide the oatmeal mixture equally into each popsicle mold. Place a popsicle stick into each and place in the freezer. Freeze at least four hours. If popsicles are reluctant to come out of their molds, dip into warm water for a few seconds. Enjoy.

Chapter 3: Protein Shakes & Smoothies

Blueberry Cacao Blast V 20

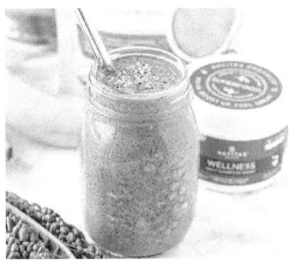

Serves: 1

Time: 5 minutes

Ingredients:

1 cup blueberries

1 tablespoon raw cacao nibs

1 tablespoon Chia seeds

1 dash cinnamon

½ Spinach (chopped)

½ Cup Bananas (chopped)

1½ Cup Almond milk

2 scoops Whey protein powder

Directions:

Place raspberries, cacao nibs, Chia seeds and cinnamon in a blender.

Add enough almond milk to reach the max line.

Process for 30 seconds or until you get a smooth mixture.

Serve immediately in the chilled tall glass.

Cucumber and Avocado Dill Smoothie V 20

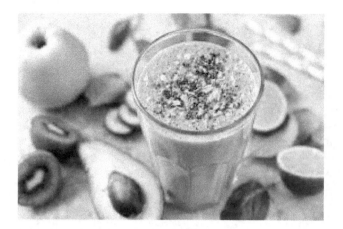

Serves: 2

Time: 5 minutes

Ingredients:

1 cucumber, peeled, sliced

2 tablespoons dill, chopped

2 tablespoons lemon juice

1 avocado, pitted

1 cup coconut milk

1 teaspoon coconut, shredded

2 kiwis, peeled, sliced

Directions

In a blender add all ingredients and blend well.

Drain the extract and discard residue.

Serve and enjoy.

Coco - Banana Milkshake V 20

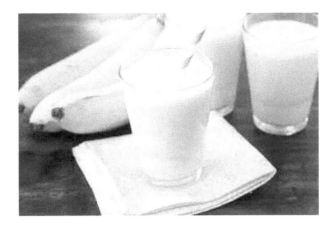

Serves: 1

Time: 5 minutes

Ingredients

1 cup coconut milk

2 ripe bananas

2 tablespoons cinnamon

¼ teaspoon cardamom powder

2 scoops protein powder

7 ice cubes

Directions

In a blender add coconut milk with cardamom powder, cinnamon, bananas and blend well.

Pour into glass and add ice chunks.

Serve and enjoy.

Stuffed Southwest Style Sweet Potatoes

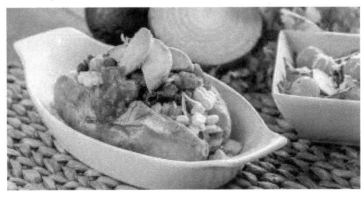

Serves: 4

Time: 60 minutes

Ingredients:

Pepper

Salt

Chopped cilantro, 2 tbs

Frozen corn kernels, ½ cup

Ground cumin, 1 tsp

Cooked black beans, ½ cup

Chopped tomatoes with juices, 1 cup

Chili powder, ½ tsp

Diced red onion, 1 small

Olive oil, 1 tsp

Small sweet potatoes, 4

Minced garlic, 1 clove

Directions:

Set your oven to 400 degrees.

Sit the sweet potatoes on a cookie sheet and allow them to bake in your heated oven for 30 minutes.

Take the potatoes out of the oven and prick them a few times and then place them back in for another 30 minutes, or until they have become tender.

As the sweet potatoes are baking, place a pan on medium heat and allow it to heat up.

Add in the olive oil and the onions and allow them to cook for two minutes. The onions should be soft, but they should not be translucent.

Add in the garlic and allow it to cook for 30 seconds or until you can start to smell the garlic.

Mix in the salt, chili powder, and cumin. Mix everything together until well combined. Mix in the cilantro and season the mixture with a bit more pepper and salt.

Taste and adjust the flavorings as you need.

To serve the potatoes:

Take the sweet potatoes out of the oven and slice them down the middle.

Fluff the meat inside of the potato up a little and season it with a bit of salt.

Divide the filling you just made between the different potatoes.

Enjoy.

Chocolate Coconut Chia Smoothie V 20

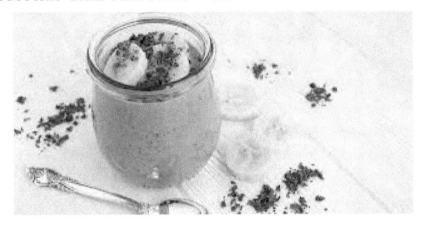

Serves: 1

Time: 5 minutes

Ingredients:

1 tablespoon raw cacao nibs

1 tablespoon Chia seeds

1 dash cinnamon

½ Spinach (chopped)

½ Cup Coconut (shredded)

1½ Cup Almond milk

Directions:

Place coconut, cacao nibs, Chia seeds and cinnamon in Vitamix.

Add enough almond milk to reach the max line.

Process for 30 seconds or until you get a smooth mixture.

Serve immediately in the tall chilled glass.

Banana-Cherry Smoothie V 20

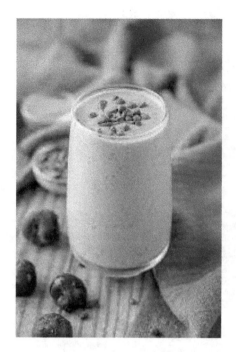

Serves: 1

Time: 5 minutes

Ingredients:

1 banana

1 cup cherries, pitted

¼ teaspoon nutmeg

1scoop protein powder

1 cup almond milk

Directions:

Place all ingredients in a blender

Process ingredients until smooth, for 20 seconds.

Serve immediately.

Avocado Smoothie V 20

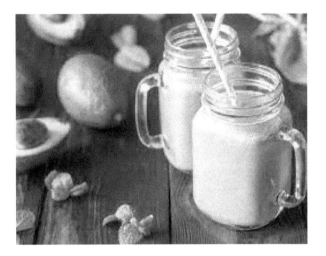

Serves: 1

Time: 5 minutes

Ingredients:

1 medium ripe avocado

¼ cup crushed peanuts

1 tablespoon flax seed

1 ½ cups vanilla Greek yogurt

1 cup Liquid (milk, water, coconut milk, etc.)

Directions:

Place all ingredients in Vitamix.

Process ingredients until smooth, for 20 seconds

Serve immediately.

Sweet Pepper Poppers

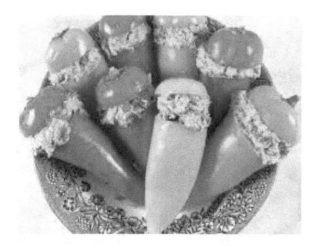

Serves: 6

Time: 20 minutes

Ingredients:

Salsa, for serving

2% shredded cheese, ½ cup

Chopped cilantro, 2 tbs

Taco seasoning packet

93% lean ground turkey, 1 pound

A bag of mini sweet bell peppers

Directions:

Start by halving the peppers and removing their seeds.

Set your oven to 350 degrees.

While the oven is heating up, brown the ground turkey.

Once the turkey is thoroughly cooked, drain off any fat that may have accumulated, and then sprinkle in the taco seasoning packet. Follow the directions on the packet for seasoning.

Place the halved bell peppers onto a baking sheet.

Ease the ground, seasoned turkey into the bell peppers.

Make sure you try to get an even amount of turkey into each bell pepper half.

Sprinkle the tops of each of the peppers with some cheese.

Place the baking tray in the oven and allow it to cook for five minutes.

Allow the peppers to cool slightly and then place over onto a serving plate. Sprinkle them with cilantro and serve them with some salsa for dipping.

Mango Smoothie V 20

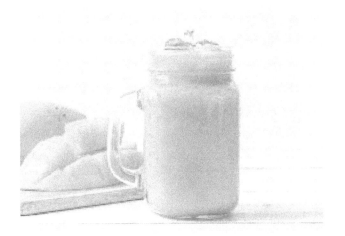

Serves: 2

Time: 5 minutes

Ingredients:

2 Mangos (seeded, diced, frozen)

Milk (1 cup)

½ cup crushed ice

1 cup plain yogurt

2 scoops protein powder

Directions:

Combine all ingredients in Vitamix.

Process for 30 seconds or until smooth

Serve immediately in a tall glass.

Pink Lady Cornmeal Cake

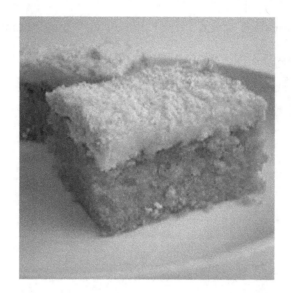

Serves: 12

Time: 1 hour 25 minutes

Ingredients:

Juice and zest of one lemon

Baking powder, 1 tsp

Ground almonds, 2 cups

Salt

Cornmeal, 1 cup

Vanilla, 1 tsp

Eggs, 3 large beaten

Splenda, ¾ cup

Butter, ⅔ cup

Pink lady apple, cored, peeled, and chopped, 1

Topping:

Pink lady apple, cored and sliced thin, 1

Confectioner's sugar, ¼ heaped cup

Zest and juice of one lemon

Crème fraîche to top

Directions:

Preheat your oven to 350 degrees. Grease and line an eight-inch round cake pan.

Place the chopped apple in a little bit of water for about six minutes until fork tender. Take off heat and drain. Let this cool.

Beat the sugar and butter together until creamy and light. Slowly mix in the eggs and beat until smooth. Mix in the baking powder, ground almonds, salt, cornmeal, and vanilla. Fold until well combined. Add in the cooled apple, lemon juice, and zest. Stir until well combined.

Carefully spoon the batter into your pan and smooth out the top. Slide into the oven for 45 minutes until golden brown and firm.

Carefully remove from oven and let it cool for around 20 minutes. Carefully turn the cake out onto a wire rack so that it can cool entirely.

While cake is cooling, make the topping. Add confectioner's sugar, four tablespoons of water, and lemon zest into a pot. Allow it to boil. Place in the sliced apples and allow it to simmer for five minutes. Spoon over the cake and let cool.

Slice into 12 even portions and serve with crème fraiche.

Bean and Spinach Burrito

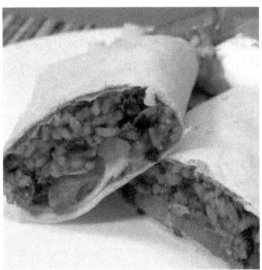

Serves: 6

Time: 30 minutes

Ingredients:

Whole grain tortillas, 6

Salt, to taste

Fat-free Greek yogurt, 6 tbs

Salsa, ½ cup

Reduced-fat grated cheddar cheese, ½ cup

Chopped romaine lettuce, ½ cup

Cooked Mexican rice, 1 ½ cups

Drained and rinsed black beans, 15 ounces

Baby spinach, 6 cups

Directions:

Set your oven to 300 degrees.

Stack all of the tortillas on top of each other and wrap them in a large piece of aluminum foil.

Sit the stack of tortillas on a baking sheet and bake them for 15 minutes until heated through.

Allow them to warm as you prepare the rest of the ingredients.

Add the spinach to the food processor and pulse it until they are finely chopped. If you don't have a food processor, you can also use a knife to slice up the leaves.

Place a large pan on medium heat and allow it to heat up.

Add in the spinach and black beans. Cook the mixture until the spinach has wilted. This should take around three minutes.

Evenly distribute this mixture between the six tortillas. Make sure that you leave about two inches on the end of the wrap to aid in folding it up.

Add about a quarter cup of the mixture to each tortilla and top with the lettuce, salsa, cheese, and the yogurt. Make sure you distribute the toppings evenly among them. Fold the tortilla over and under on the ends.

Cilantro Lime Cauliflower Rice

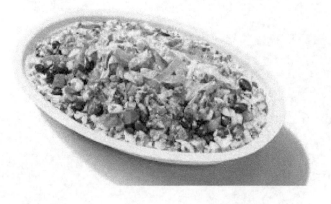

Serves: 4

Time: 6 minutes

Ingredients:

Chopped cilantro, 1 ½ tbs

Sea salt, ¼ tsp

Fresh lime juice, 1 tbs

Frozen riced cauliflower, 10 oz

Directions:

Follow the directions on the package of riced cauliflower to cook it.

As the cauliflower is cooking, chop up your cilantro.

Take the cauliflower out of the microwave and open the bag to allow all of the steam to release. Make sure that you don't get burned.

Pour the cooked cauliflower into a bowl and add in the salt, cilantro, and lime juice. Stir everything together to combine all of the flavors.

Chicken Curry

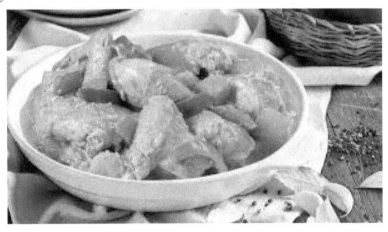

Serves: 4

Time: 60 minutes

Ingredients:

Cornmeal, 2 tbs

Cilantro, chopped, 2 tbs

Chicken stock, ¾ cup

Light coconut milk, 14 ounces

Sweet potato, 7 ounces peeled and chopped

Granny Smith apple that has been peeled, cored, and chopped, 1

Chicken breast, skinless, boneless, 1 pound, cut into cubes

Cinnamon stick

Cardamom pods, 6, crushed

Ground cumin, 1 tsp

Turmeric, 1 tsp

Red chili that has been seeded and chopped, 1

Garlic cloves, 2 crushed

One large onion that has been chopped

Low-fat cooking spray

Directions:

Coat a skillet with nonstick spray. Warm up the skillet on the burner and then add the onion and garlic, cooking until soft. This should take about five minutes. Place in the cinnamon stick, cardamom pods, cumin, turmeric, and chili and cook for an additional two minutes.

Place chicken into skillet and cook for three minutes. Stir to combine everything. Add cilantro, chicken stock, coconut milk, sweet potato, and apple. Stir well again. Partially cover the skillet and turn the heat down to a simmer. Let this cook for 35 minutes. Add water as needed.

Mix the cornmeal with a small amount of water. Mix together. Add to chicken mixture. Stir well until mixture is slightly thickened.

Serve hot over rice if desired.

Corn and Black Bean Salad

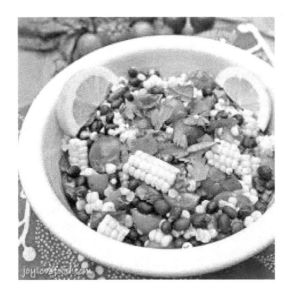

Serves: 30

Time: 6 minutes

Ingredients

Pepper, ¼ tsp

Olive oil, 2 tbs

Dash of salt

Brown sugar or honey, 1 tsp

Minced garlic, 1 tsp

Balsamic vinegar, ¼ cup

Minced red onion, 2 tbs

Chopped parsley, ¼ cup

Drained and rinsed black beans, 2, 16-ounce cans

Whole kernel corn, 1 cup

Directions:

Place the parsley, red onion, black beans, and corn in a large bowl and mix everything together.

Whisk the pepper, salt, honey, garlic, lemon juice, olive oil, and balsamic vinegar together. Make sure that all of the seasonings are mixed together well.

Pour the dressing you just made over the corn and bean mixture.

Toss everything together and allow the vegetables to marinate for at least 30 minutes before you serve them.

This will allow all of the flavors to mix together, and the flavor will be a lot more intense.

Enjoy.

Chicken Nuggets

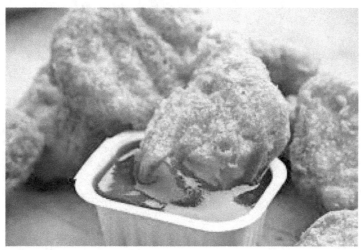

Serves: 4

Time: 50 minutes

Ingredients

2 tbsp. parmesan

3 tsp. canola oil

Nonstick spray

1 lb. chicken breasts, diced

3 tbsp. panko breadcrumbs

½ tsp. salt

¼ tsp. oregano

½ tsp. Italian herbs

¼ tsp. pepper

½ tsp. garlic salt

Directions

Heat your oven to 450.

Coat the chicken with oil. Sprinkle with pepper, garlic salt, oregano, salt, and Italian herbs. Massage into each piece of chicken.

Put the breadcrumbs and parmesan cheese into a gallon zippered bag and add the chicken. Seal the bag and shake and squeeze the chicken to coat it well.

Spray cooking spray on a cookie sheet.

Put chicken nugget in a single layer on the cookie sheet.

Spritz the chicken with some cooking spray.

Place in the oven and cook for eight minutes until no longer pink.

Chia Blueberry Banana Oatmeal Smoothie V 20

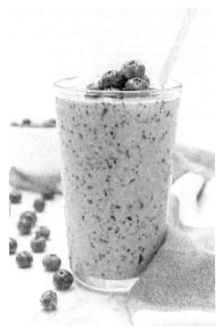

Serves: 1

Time: 10m

Ingredients:

Soy milk (1 cups)

Frozen banana (1, sliced)

Frozen blueberries (1/4 cup)

Oats (1/4 cup)

Vanilla extract (1 tsp.)

Cinnamon (1 tsp., to taste)

Chia seed (1 tbs.)

Directions:

Add all ingredients into a blender and blend until the ingredients are combined and smooth.

Serve and enjoy!

Strawberry and Cherry Shake V 20

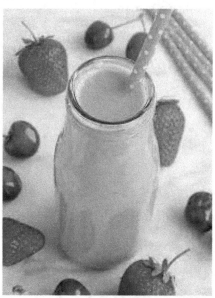

Serves: 2

Time: 5 minutes

Ingredients:

1 cup strawberries

1 cup cherries

1 cup almond milk

½ cup coconut milk

2 scoops protein powder

Few ice chunks

Directions

In a blender add all ingredients and blend well.

Serve and enjoy.

Pineapple Shake V 20

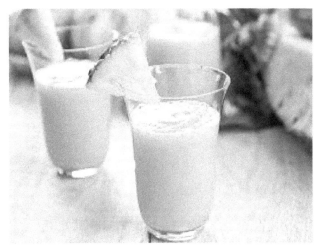

Serves: 6

Time: 20 minutes

Ingredients:

Frozen pineapple (3 cups)

Whey Protein Powder (2 scoops)

Greek yogurt (1 cup, pineapple/vanilla flavored)

Unsweetened vanilla almond milk (1 cup)

Vanilla extract (1 tbs.)

Directions:

Add the ingredients in the blender and blend until smooth.

Serve and enjoy!

Spicy Peanut Vegetarian Chili

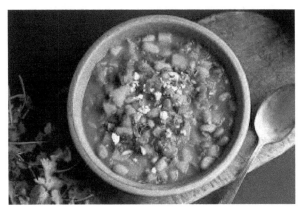

Serves: 12

Time: 50 minutes

Ingredients:

Vegetable broth, 2 cups

Tomato sauce, 15 ounces

Diced tomato, 28 ounces

Powdered peanuts, ⅔ cup

Rinsed and drained white beans, 16 ounces

Rinsed and drained, black beans, 16 ounces

Dried oregano, ¼ tsp

Chipotle chili pepper, 1 tsp (optional)

Chili powder, 2 tbs

Minced garlic, 2 cloves

Chopped onion, 1 cup

Peanut oil, 1 tbs

Directions:

In a Dutch oven, pour the oil in and let it heat up over medium-high heat.

Place in the onion and garlic and sauté them together for three to four minutes. The onions should become tender, but make sure that you don't let your garlic burn.

Mix in the salt, oregano, pepper, and chili powder. Allow this mixture to sauté for another two minutes, or until it becomes fragrant.

Mix in the broth, tomato sauce, tomatoes, powdered peanuts, corn, and cleaned beans.

Stir everything together and let it all come to a boil.

Lower the heat down to a simmer and allow the mixture to cook for 30 minutes.

If you want, this can also be fixed in a slow cooker.

Add everything to the slow cooker and mix everything together.

Cover the slow cooker and set it to high for two to three hours.

Halloumi Wraps

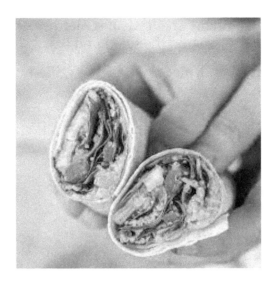

Serves: 6

Time: 30 minutes

Ingredients

Dressing:

1 olive oil

2 tbsp. sweet chili sauce

Filling and Salad:

6 radishes, sliced

9 oz. Halloumi cheese

4 spring onions, sliced

4 wraps, low-carb

1 head lettuce, leaves separated

1 lime, juiced

2 celery stalks, sliced

Directions

Combine the dressing ingredients and stir well to combine.

Slice the Halloumi into eight equal slices and coat with the dressing.

Put them on the grill or in a pan and brown on both sides about three minutes. They need to be crispy and browned on the outside.

While these are cooking, combine the radishes, lettuce, spring onions, and celery together. Add the rest of the dressing on the salad and toss.

Divide this between the wraps and place two of the grilled cheese slices on each. Serve immediately.

Enjoy.

Sichuan Roasted Eggplant

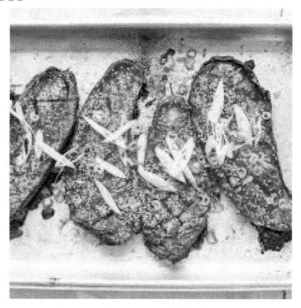

Serves: 4

Time: 80 minutes

Ingredients

1 tbsp. dark soy sauce

4 cloves crushed garlic

3 eggplants

2 tbsp. tomato paste

Pepper

3 tsp. chopped ginger

2 tbsp. olive oil

1 red chili, chopped finely

Salt

2 tbsp. sweet chili sauce

2 tsp. honey

Optional Toppings

Sesame oil

6 spring onions, chopped

Directions

Set your oven to 400. Put foil or silicone pad on a baking sheet. To make cleanup easier.

Mix pepper, ginger, honey, chili, salt, sweet chili sauce, tomato paste, oil, and soy sauce.

Slice eggplants in half lengthwise and make deep crisscross scores into the eggplants. Don't cut through the skins. Mark the flesh only. Put eggplants on the baking sheet and spoon the paste you made earlier on the flesh. Cover the eggplants loosely with foil and cook for about 30 minutes.

Remove the foil and allow to cook for another 30 minutes. They need to be brown and tender. Drizzle with some sesame oil and let stand for five minutes.

Top with chopped onions.

Enjoy.

Crustless Pizza Bites

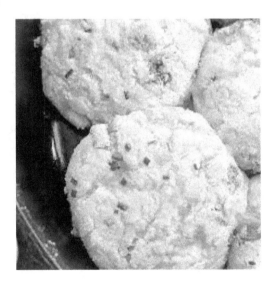

Serves: 5

Time: 45 minutes

Ingredients

Shredded mozzarella cheese

Pizza toppings of choice

Thick cut Canadian bacon

Pizza sauce

Directions

Spray cooking spray in a regular muffin tin. Put three slices of Canadian bacon in the bottom of each cup. Let the overlap to look like a three-leaf clover. Press down to form them to the cups. They don't like to stay well, but it's okay. When you put the toppings in, they will stay.

Get your cheese, sauce, and toppings together.

Put one tablespoon pizza sauce in each cup.

Add whatever toppings you would like that the cups will hold.

Sprinkle with a good amount of mozzarella cheese.

Heat your oven to 350. Put the pizzas in the oven for 27 minutes or until browned and bubbly. Watch them closely, so they don't burn.

Remove the pizzas from the pan with a fork. There will be some liquid in the bottom of the muffin cups, just throw away and enjoy your pizza bites.

Thai Sea Bass

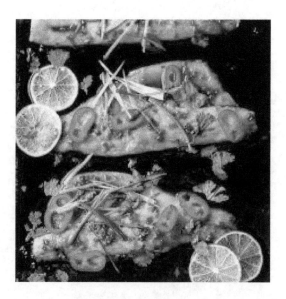

Serves: 5

Time: 20 minutes

Ingredients

2 tbsp. chopped cilantro

8 oz. bok choy, quartered

1 tbsp. soy sauce

4 oz. asparagus, trimmed

2 sea bass fillets

2 spring onions, chopped

Zest and juice of one lemon

1 mild red chili, sliced and seeded

2 cloves crushed garlic

4 tsp. grated ginger

1 tbsp. fish sauce

3 tbsp. oil

Directions

Heat your oven to 400.

Place the onions, bok choy, and asparagus in a roasting pan.

Mix lemon juice, fish sauce, garlic, lemon zest, chili, oil, soy sauce, and ginger together. Pour half over the vegetables and toss to coat. Slide this into the oven and cook for five minutes.

Take the veggies out and put the sea bass on top. Put back into the oven for another eight minutes until fish is cooked through. It should flake when you poke it with a fork.

Pour remaining dressing on top of fish, top with cilantro and enjoy.

Pacific Cod with Fajita Vegetables (Dairy-Free)

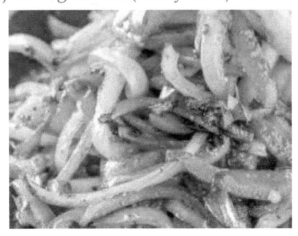

Serves: 4

Time: 20 minutes

Ingredients:

Pepper

Salt

Large julienned carrot, 1

Sliced yellow bell pepper, 2

Sliced red bell pepper, 2

Low-fat nonstick spray

Scallions, 6

Juice and zest of a lime

Wild Alaskan Pacific cod, 4, 6-ounce fillets

Directions:

Heat up your grill or broiler.

Place some aluminum foil over the grill rack and place the cod fillets on top.

Top the fillets with the lime juice, zest, and some slices of the scallions.

Allow them to grill or broil for six to eight minutes, or until it is cooked all the way through. The fish will turn opaque and will easily flake once it is cooked through.

As the fish cooks, spray a large skillet with some low-fat nonstick spray and allow it to heat up for a few moments on high.

Add in the bell peppers, the rest of the scallions, and carrot.

Allow them to cook, stirring often, for three to five minutes.

Divide your cooked veggies between four different plates and top each of them with a cod fillet.

Season the top of the fish with some pepper and salt to taste.

Mini Meatloaves

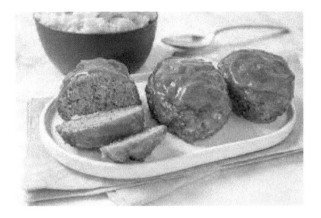

Serves: 4

Time: 50 minutes

Ingredients

¼ c whole wheat panko breadcrumbs

¾ c reduced fat shredded cheese

½ c chopped green bell pepper

¼ c egg whites

1 tsp. garlic powder

¼ tsp. pepper

3 tbsp. ketchup

½ tsp. salt

1 c chopped onion

1 tsp. onion powder

1 lb. ground beef

1 tsp. mustard

Optional Toppings:

Ketchup

Mustard

Dill pickles

Directions

Heat your oven to 375. Spray cooking spray in a regular muffin tin.

Stir together all of the ingredients, except for the cheese and toppings. Everything needs to be combined well. Divide the meat evenly among the cups and smooth out the tops.

Bake for 35 minutes until edges are browned and the meatloaf is firm.

Sprinkle with the cheese and cook for another three minutes until the cheese is melted and browned.

Take the dish from the oven and take out of the muffin pan with a knife or fork. Serve with toppings of choice and enjoy.

Salmon with Summer Salsa (Dairy-Free)

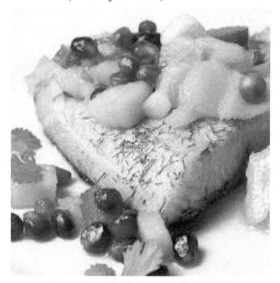

Serves: 4

Time: 55 minutes

Ingredients:

Lime wedges

Chopped cilantro, ¼ cup

Pepper

Balsamic vinegar, 1 tbs

Salt

Minced red onion, ¼ cup

Cooked corn kernels, ½ cup

Olive oil, 1 tsp

Crushed garlic clove

Chopped avocado, ½ an avocado

Chopped tomato, 1 cup

Skinless salmon, 4, 4-ounce fillets

Directions:

Set your oven to 325 degrees.

Stir all of the ingredients together, except for the lime and salmon.

Allow the mixture to refrigerate for around 30 minutes so that all of the flavors can meld together.

Place the salmon in your preheated oven and let it cook for 15 to 20 minutes, or until it has cooked all the way through. The salmon should flake easily and should be opaque when it is fully cooked.

Serve the cooked salmon topped with the salsa and lime wedge. A great summer option is to allow the salmon to cool off completely after it has cooked. Serving cool salmon with the chilled salsa is delicious.

Roasted Corn Guacamole

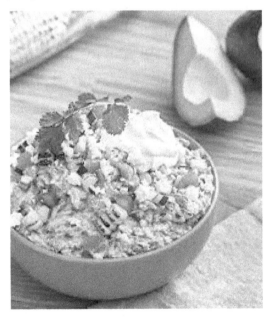

Serves: 6

Time: 15 minutes

Ingredients:

Pepper

Salt

Chili pepper, 1 tsp

Garlic powder, 1 ½ tsp

Chopped cilantro, ¼ cup

Diced onion, ¼ cup

Diced small tomato

Lime juice, 2 tsp

Large avocados, 2-3

Cumin, 2 tsp, divided

Butter, 1 tbs

An ear of corn

Directions:

Heat up a grill. Brush the corn with some butter and sprinkle it with a teaspoon of the cumin.

Lay the corn on the grill and cook it for five minutes. Make sure you turn it often during the cooking process to make sure it browns evenly.

The corn should char slightly during the cooking process.

Take it off the grill, and with a sharp knife, slice off the kernels. Set the kernels aside and discard the cob.

Pit the avocados and scoop out the meat of the avocados and place it in a bowl.

Mash up the avocados using a fork until they are creamy, but they still have a little bit of texture.

Mix in the garlic powder, chili powder, cilantro, and lime juice. Mix all of the ingredients together to make sure everything is evenly distributed.

Add in some pepper and salt to taste. Carefully stir in the corn, tomatoes, and onion.

Serve the guacamole immediately.

This is a great topper for any of the recipes in the beef and poultry sections of this book.

Spinach Green Smoothie V 20

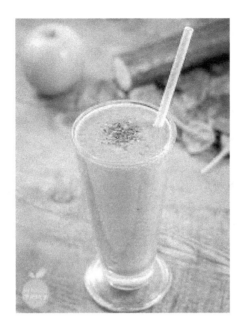

Serves: 2

Time: 5 min

Ingredients:

1 cup baby spinach leaves

2-3 mint leave

1 cup 100% grapes juice

1 cup 100% pineapple juice

2 tablespoons lime juice

2 scoops protein powder

Directions

In a blender add ingredients and blend well till puree.

Transfer to serving glasses.

Serve and enjoy.

Vegetable Chili

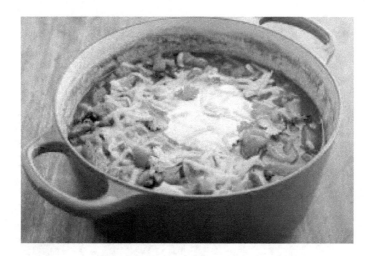

Serves: 12

Time: 8 hours 15 minutes

Ingredients:

Cilantro, ½ cup

Corn kernels, 1 cup

Vegetable broth, 2 ½ cups

Tomato paste, 6 ounces

Diced green chilis, 4 ounces

Cumin, 1 tsp

Drained black beans, 2 cans

Diced tomatoes, 2, 15-ounce cans

Salt, 1 tsp

Pepper, ½ tsp

Diced sweet potato

Diced celery, 1 cup

Diced sweet onion, 1 cup

Chili powder, 3 tbs

Sliced carrots, 2 cups

Dark red kidney beans, 1 can

Directions:

Place all of the chili ingredients, except for the cilantro, into a slow cooker.

Stir everything together and place the lid on the cooker and then set it to cook for six to eight hours on low.

Once it has finished cooking, sprinkle in the cilantro. You can also top the chili with some diced avocado, sour cream, and shredded cheese.

Black Bean, Rice, and Zucchini Skillet

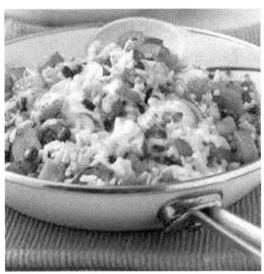

Serves: 4

Time: 25 minutes

Ingredients:

Monterey Jack and Cheddar cheese blend, shredded, ½ cup

Uncooked instant white rice, 1 cup

Dried oregano, ¼ tsp

Water, ¾ cup

Undrained fire roasted diced tomatoes with garlic, 14.5 ounces

Rinsed and drained black beans, 15 ounces

Diced green bell pepper, ½ cup

Chopped onion, ½ cup

Small sliced zucchini

Canola oil, 1 tbs

Directions:

Start out by heating the oil in a large pan over medium heat.

Once it is well heated, add in the bell pepper, zucchini, and onion. Allow the veggies to cook for five minutes, or until softened.

Make sure that you stir them occasionally.

Add in the oregano, water, undrained tomatoes, and beans.

Bring the heat up a bit and allow it to come to a boil.

Mix in the rice, stirring well to distribute all of the flavors.

Place the lid on the pan and then set it off the heat.

Allow the mixture to sit for seven minutes, or until the rice has absorbed all of the water.

Sprinkle everything with cheese and enjoy.

Mini Chicken Parmesan

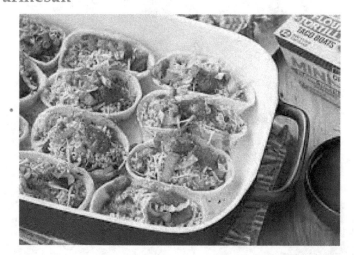

Serves: 4

Time: 35 minutes

Ingredients

1 egg

¾ c pasta sauce

1 ½ lb. ground chicken breast

¾ c mozzarella cheese, reduced fat

1 egg white

2 cloves minced garlic

6 tbsp. breadcrumbs

¾ c parmesan cheese

¾ tsp. dried basil

1/3 tsp. pepper

¾ tsp. oregano

¾ tsp. dried thyme

½ small chopped onion

¾ tsp. salt

Directions

Heat the oven to 350. Spray cooking spray into a muffin tin.

Mix the parmesan, pepper, egg, onion, salt, egg whites, garlic, oregano, breadcrumbs, thyme, basil, and chicken. Don't overmix. Make sure all the ingredients are distributed throughout the chicken.

Divide the mixture evenly into the muffin cups. Put pasta sauce over the meat mixture. Slide this in the oven for 20 minutes. Remove from the oven and add one tablespoon shredded cheese. Put back in the oven to let the cheese melt.

Take out of the muffin pan with a knife and enjoy.

Stuffed Chicken

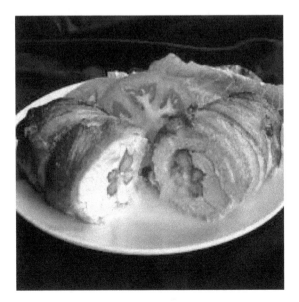

Serves: 4

Time: 40 minutes

Ingredients

Pepper

4 chicken cutlets, pounded thin

Salt

½ c breadcrumbs

Tomato sauce

¼ c parmesan, divided

Mozzarella cheese

1 egg

½ c ricotta cheese

½ pack frozen spinach, thawed and well drained

Directions

Heat your oven to 425.

Add half the breadcrumbs and parmesan cheese to a bowl, mix to combine. Set to the side.

Squeeze the spinach to get rid of all the liquid in it. Mix the rest of the parmesan with the ricotta and spinach in a bowl.

Put the cutlet on a cutting board and spread two tablespoons of the spinach on the top.

Roll up and secure with toothpicks.

In a shallow dish, whisk the eggs.

Coat each cutlet with egg and then the breadcrumbs.

Place them seam side down in a baking dish that you prepared with nonstick spray. Slide this in the oven for 25 minutes.

Take this out and top with some tomato sauce and mozzarella cheese.

Slide this back into the oven for five more minutes.

Remove from the oven and enjoy.

Fajita Chicken

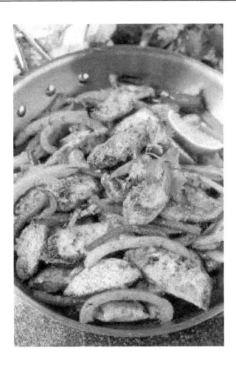

Serves: 4

Time: 8 hours 10 minutes

Ingredients

1 bag frozen pepper and onion blend

1 packet taco seasoning

Garlic powder

3 lb. frozen boneless chicken breast

3 c chunky salsa

Directions

Place the frozen chicken into a Crock-Pot. Sprinkle with taco seasoning and spoon salsa on each one. Sprinkle with garlic powder then add frozen onions and pepper on top.

Place the lid on and set on low for eight hours.

Serve as it is or shred for tacos, nachos, taco salad, fajitas, burritos or add to a baked potato. Leftovers can be stored in the refrigerator for a week or frozen.

Lamb Koftas

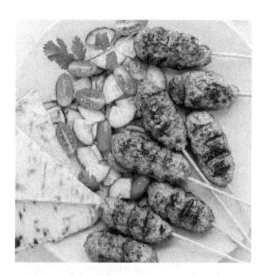

Serves: 4

Time: 40 minutes

Ingredients

2 tbsp. mint, chopped

8 oz. lean ground lamb

2 tbsp. fat-free dressing

2 tbsp. chopped parsley

2 oz. bulgur wheat

4 oz. light feta cheese

½ small chopped onion

8 oz. cherry tomatoes, halved

1 clove crushed garlic

½ cucumber, sliced and halved

½ tsp. cumin

½ tsp. ground coriander

1 ½ oz. craisins

Directions

Put the wheat into a skillet then cover with water and allow to boil. Cook for five minutes. The wheat needs to be tender then drain completely.

Combine garlic, lamb, onion, and wheat together. Mix the parsley, cumin, craisins, and coriander. Stir until all is incorporated. Divide the meat into 12 even portions.

Set your oven to broil or warm up a grill. Take one portion of the meat and press it around a skewer to form an oval. Continue with the remaining portions. Put them on a broiler pan or grill. Cook for about ten minutes. Turn about halfway through to brown both sides.

While the meat is cooking, combine parsley, cucumbers, mint, tomatoes, and feta. Toss in the dressing. Serve with the koftas.

Vegetable Chili

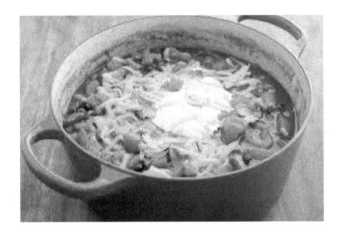

Serves: 3

Time: 20 minutes

Ingredients

1 tsp. chopped rosemary

7 oz. Romano peppers, seeded and sliced

1 red onion, sliced

Cilantro - garnish

14 oz. black beans, drained and rinsed

½ c strong low-fat grated cheese

12 oz. cherry tomato and basil sauce

2 tsp. chipotle paste

Cooking spray

Directions

Coat a pan generously with nonstick spray. Allow it to heat up and add the rosemary, peppers, and red onion. Cook for five minutes.

Add the chipotle paste, beans, and cherry tomato and basil sauce. Allow to simmer for about ten minutes. The peppers need to be tender.

Serve with some grated cheese and cilantro.

Enjoy.

Beef and Broccoli Stir-Fry

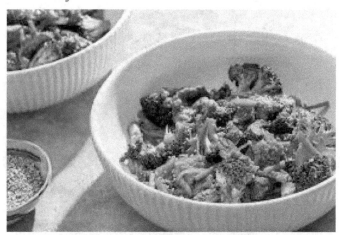

Serves: 4

Time: 50 minutes

Ingredients

1 tsp. rice vinegar

1 tsp. ginger, grated

4 scallions, shredded

4 tbsp. oyster sauce

12 oz. beef steak, cut into 1/2 -inch strips

2 red chilies, thinly sliced

Cooking spray

5 oz. shiitake mushrooms, sliced

1 tbsp. light soy sauce

1 red thickly sliced onion

8 oz. broccoli, cut in half

Directions

Combine the soy sauce and ginger and add the steak and coat well. Allow to sit for 15 minutes.

Use cooking spray to coat a wok then allow to heat up. When hot, place the steak mixture. Stir-fry the steak for five minutes until browned. Put the steak in a bowl for later use.

Put chili, broccoli, mushrooms, and onion in the wok and cook for about five minutes until veggies are tender. Add water or more cooking spray, so food doesn't burn.

Put the steak along with its juices back into the wok and add the rice vinegar and oyster sauce. Stir to combine. Cook a few minutes more until everything is heated through.

Garnish with scallions. Enjoy.

Spicy Peanut Vegetarian Chili

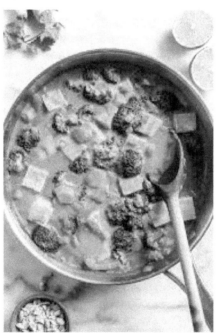

Serves: 4

Time: 50 minutes

Ingredients

2 c vegetable broth

¼ tsp. dried oregano

1 16 oz. can white beans, drained and rinsed

1 c chopped onion

1 15 oz. can tomato sauce

1 can black beans, drained and rinsed

2 tbsp. chili powder

1 28 oz. can diced tomatoes

2/3 c powdered peanuts

1 tsp. chipotle chili powder

1 tbsp. peanut oil

2 cloves minced garlic

Directions

Add oil to a Dutch oven and allow to heat up. Add the onion and garlic then sauté until tender and fragrant. Add the salt, chili powder, oregano, and pepper. Cook for another two minutes. Add the broth, beans, tomato sauce, corn, tomatoes, and powdered peanuts. Allow to boil then reduce the heat and simmer for 30 minutes.

Spoon into serving bowls and enjoy.

Chicken and Vegetables

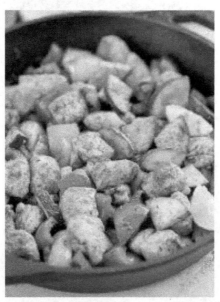

Serves: 6

Time: 50 minutes

Ingredients

4 yellow or red sliced bell peppers

3 to 4 cloves minced garlic

2 small diced Vidalia onions

1 8 oz. can tomato sauce

3 small zucchini, sliced

3 16 oz. cans diced tomatoes

8 oz. sliced mushrooms

3 lb. bag boneless skinless chicken breast

Directions

Cut the chicken into cubes. Put into a large pan along with the garlic and onion. Cook until almost done.

Add the tomato sauce, bell peppers, canned tomatoes, zucchini, and mushrooms. Cover and allow to cook for about 20 minutes. The vegetables need to be tender then taste to see if you need more pepper and salt

Serve over rice or as it is. Store leftovers in the refrigerator for one week or can be frozen to be eaten later.

Taco Chicken

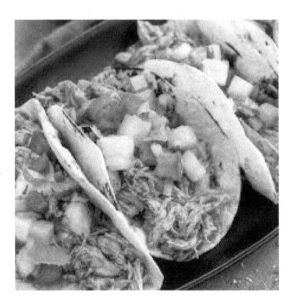

Serves: 2

Time: 40 minutes

Ingredients

1 c salsa

1 packet taco seasoning

¼ c nonfat sour cream

4 4 oz. chicken breast

Directions

Heat your oven to 375.

Put the taco seasoning in a reseal-able bag. Place the chicken and shake to coat. Place the chicken in a baking dish that is greased with nonstick spray. Bake for 30 minutes but take out of the oven at 25 minutes and top with salsa. Place back in the oven and bake for five more minutes. Remove from the oven and top with sour cream. Serve as it is or shred for tacos. Enjoy.

Vegetable Stir-Fry

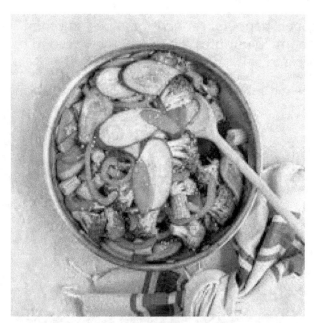

Serves: 5

Time: 25 minutes

Ingredients

1 chili, finely chopped

4 tbsp. soy sauce

2 red peppers, sliced and cored

1 onion, sliced

11 oz. baby corn, halved

1 lb. oriental mushrooms

2 tsp. sesame oil

2 cloves crushed garlic

1 lb. Chinese leaf lettuce, shredded

Cilantro for Garnish

Directions

Put oil in a wok and heat it.

Place the garlic and chili and let cook for 30 seconds.

Add the peppers, mushrooms, Chinese lettuce, and corn. Stir-fry for four minutes until they are tender-crisp.

Pour soy sauce over everything and toss to coat.

Serve garnished with cilantro.

Black Bean and Turkey Sloppy Joes

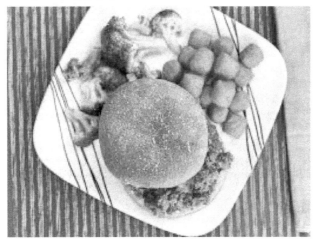

Serves: 4

Time: 70 minutes

Ingredients

1 14 oz. can diced tomatoes with green chilies

1 tsp. minced garlic

1 tsp. Mrs. Dash onion and herb blend

1 lb. ground turkey

1 6 oz. can tomato paste

1 14 oz. can black beans, drained and rinsed

1 ½ c low sodium tomato juice

1 tsp. paprika

1 tbsp. olive oil

1 medium chopped onion

2 tsp. chili powder

Directions

Put the turkey into a skillet and brown then drain any fat. Put all of the ingredients into the skillet and cook until the desired thickness.

Serve on buns or over toast.

Lemon Chicken Kebabs

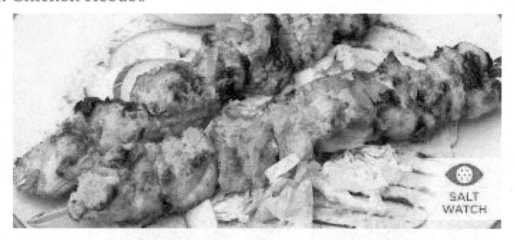

Serves: 4

Time: 55 minutes

Ingredients

2 tbsp. olive oil

Vegetables such as tomatoes and zucchini

2 lemons, juiced

1 tbsp. lemon zest

4 chicken breasts, cubed

Dipping Sauce:

2 cloves crushed garlic

Zest and juice of ½ lemon

3 tbsp. chopped basil

8 oz. plain goat cheese yogurt

Garnish:

2 tsp. basil

Directions

Put lemon juice, oil, pepper, salt, and lemon zest in a bowl and mix together well. Place the chicken and coat well. Cover the bowl and allow to marinate about 30 minutes.

While this marinates, combine the yogurt, pepper, garlic, lemon juice, salt, lemon zest, and basil in a bowl to make the dipping sauce. Put in the refrigerator until needed.

Thread the vegetables and the chicken onto eight to 12 skewers. Make sure you alternate them. Grill kebabs about five minutes per side. Turn them often, so they don't burn. As they cook, baste them with leftover marinade.

When chicken is done, serve with dipping sauce. Garnish with basil.

Enjoy.

Chapter 4: Veggies and Fruits

Black Bean and Rice Casserole

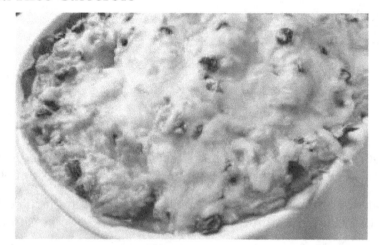

Serves: 8

Time: 90 minutes

Ingredients

1 cup vegetable broth

1/3 cup each:

Diced onion

Brown rice

1 tablespoon olive oil

1 lb. chopped chicken breast (no skin or bones)

1 medium thinly sliced zucchini

½ cup sliced mushrooms

¼ teaspoon cayenne pepper

½ teaspoon cumin

1/3 cup shredded carrots

1 can (4 ounces) diced green chilies

1 can (15 ounces) drained black beans

2 cups shredded Swiss cheese

Directions

Prepare a pot with the vegetable broth and rice, bringing it to a boil. Lower the heat setting and cook covered on low for 45 minutes.

Program the oven temperature to 350°F.

Spray a baking dish with some cooking spray.

Pour the oil in a pan over medium heat. Toss in the onion and cook until tender, and blend in the chicken, zucchini, mushrooms, and seasonings. Continue cooking until the chicken is heated and the zucchini is lightly browned.

In a large mixing dish, combine the onion, cooked rice, chicken, zucchini, beans, chilies, mushrooms, one cup of Swiss cheese, and the carrots.

Empty the ingredients into the casserole dish along with the remainder of the Swiss cheese as a topping. Cover and bake 30 minutes. Uncover, and continue cooking ten more minutes.

Broccoli Casserole

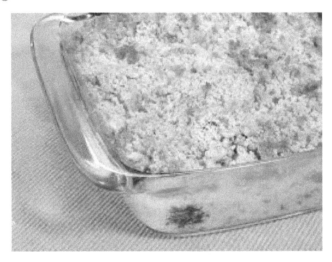

Serves: 12

Time: 50 minutes

Ingredients

4 cups cut up broccoli

1 sleeve Ritz crackers

2 cups cheddar cheese

Directions

Add the casserole ingredients into a Pyrex dish with the crumbled crackers on top.

Bake long enough to melt the cheese at 375°F.

Veggies with Grilled Pineapple

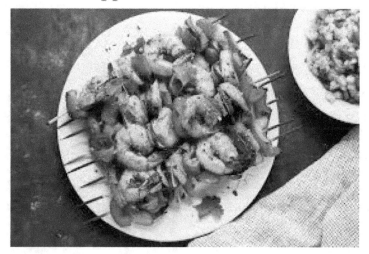

Serves: 6

Time: 40 minutes

Ingredients

1 cup of each:

Diced potatoes

Bell peppers

Raw mushrooms

1 cup cherry tomatoes

1 medium chopped onion

1 can of pineapple chunks – natural juices

2 teaspoons each:

Dill weed

Chopped garlic

1 teaspoon celery seed/salt

3 tablespoons olive oil

1 ½ teaspoons each: **Optional**:

Onion powder

Cayenne pepper

Garlic powder

Pepper and salt to taste

Directions

Chop the veggies

Option 1: Add the veggies on a piece of oil sprayed foil. Arrange the package on the grill using medium heat for 20-25 minutes (turning every five minutes).

Option 2: Place the veggies on wooden skewers that have been soaked in water. Cook on a med-high grill, turning every five minutes or so.

Oven: Bake at 400ºF, checking every 10 minutes.

Vegetarian Frittata

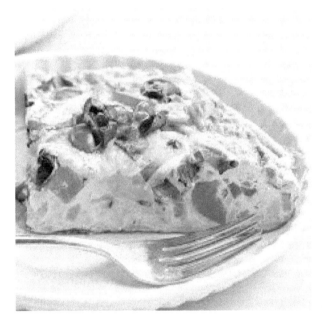

Serves: 6

Time: 60 minutes

Ingredients

6 ounces button mushrooms

1 pound asparagus

1 shallot

1 garlic clove

1 tablespoon olive oil

1 small zucchini

6 large eggs

1/3 cup 1% milk

¼ teaspoon of freshly ground black pepper

1 teaspoon salt

1 tablespoon chopped chives

Dash of nutmeg

2 medium/1 large tomato

¼ cup freshly grated parmesan cheese

Directions

Set the oven temperature to 350°F.

Prepare the Asparagus: Wash and trim cutting it into one-inch pieces. Blanche the cut asparagus for one to two minutes. Shock it by adding it to ice water. Drain and set to the side.

Wash and slice the mushrooms. Saute them in the oil for ten minutes using medium heat. Mince the shallots and garlic and add – cooking two more minutes. Transfer the mushrooms to a plate and set aside.

Slice the zucchini lengthwise and into half-moon shapes.

Whisk the eggs, milk, chives, pepper, salt, and nutmeg in a large mixing dish. Add the mushroom mixture, asparagus, and zucchini.

Spray a two-quart baking dish with cooking spray and add the egg/veggie mixture.

Arrange the thinly sliced tomatoes on top and sprinkle with the parmesan cheese.

Bake 30-35 minutes. You can place the frittata under the broiler for two to three minutes to brown the top.

Cool and serve at room temperature or straight from the fridge.

Chickpea and Feta Salad

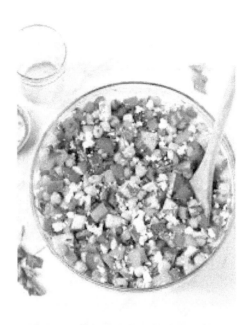

Serves: 1

Time: 55 minutes

Ingredients

¾ cup chopped raw vegetables

¼ cup each:

Can/fresh chickpeas

Crumbled feta cheese

1 tablespoon lemon juice

2 tablespoons olive oil

1 teaspoon dried oregano

Dash each of:

Pepper

Salt

Directions

Use your imagination for the chopped veggies. Include peppers, avocado, tomatoes, onions, and celery or your favorites.

Rinse and drain the chickpeas.

Combine all of the ingredients and chill in the fridge until ready to serve.

Cucumber and Onion Salad with Vinegar

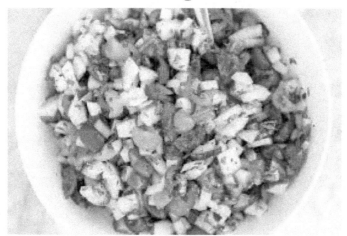

Serves: 6

Time: 70 minutes

Ingredients

Pinch of salt and pepper

1 red onion

3-5 cucumbers (peeled)

½ cup each:

White vinegar

Water

1/3 cup sugar

Directions

Slice the cucumbers and onions very thin and add to a salad dish.

Combine the water, vinegar, salt, pepper, and sugar and pour over the veggies.

Add a cover and marinate for a minimum of one hour.

Coleslaw

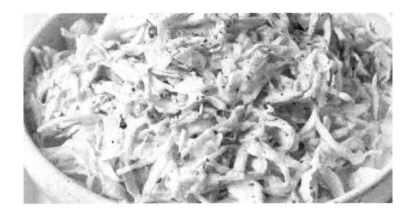

Serves: 6

Time: 35 minutes

Ingredients

1 small shredded carrot

3 cups green cabbage – shredded

¼ cup minced onion

1 tablespoon vinegar

1/3 cup mayonnaise

2 teaspoons sugar

½ teaspoon each:

Celery seed

Salt

Directions

Prepare the onion, carrots, and cabbage into a bowl.

Mix the dressing and pour over the slaw.

Lentil Vegetarian Loaf

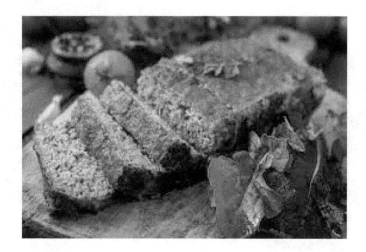

Serves: 10

Time: 2 hours 20 minutes

Ingredients

1 ½ cups rinsed – dried lentils

2 yellow onions

3 cups cooked brown rice

2 tablespoons canola/olive oil

½ cup ketchup

1 can tomato paste (6 ounces)

1 teaspoon each of:

Marjoram

Garlic powder

Sage

½ cup - quartered cherry tomatoes

¾ cup tomato/pasta sauce

To Taste:

Salt

More ketchup

Directions

Preheat the oven to 350°F.

Rinse and cook the lentils in 3 to 4 cups of water for approximately 30 minutes.

Drain and slightly mash the lentils.

Peel and chop the onions. Cook in the oil until golden.

Combine the onions, lentils, tomato paste, rice, tomatoes, sauce and spices into a large pot. Mix well.

Press the mixture into a well-greased baking dish with ½ cup of ketchup over the top.

Bake for one hour.

Baked Tomatoes

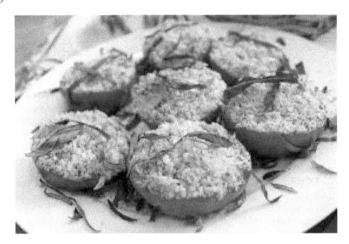

Serves: 6

Time: 60 minutes

Ingredients

Olive oil spray

5-6 large tomatoes

Greek seasoning

¼ cup low-fat parmesan cheese

Optional: ¼ cup pine nuts

Directions

Set the oven temperature in advance to 350°F. Spray a baking pan with the olive oil.

Slice the tomatoes lengthwise into halves and arrange them on the baking pan.

Sprinkle them with the cheese, nuts, and a bit of Greek seasoning as you desire.

Bake on the middle oven rack for 50 minutes.

Acorn Squash- Stuffed with Cheese

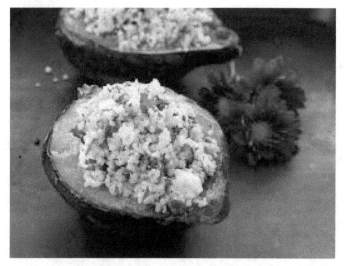

Serves: 4

Time: 60 minutes

Ingredients

1 pound ground turkey breast (extra-lean)

2 acorn squash

1 can (8 ounces) tomato sauce

1 cup each:

Sliced fresh mushrooms

Chopped onion

Diced celery

1 teaspoon each:

Garlic powder

Basil

Oregano

1 pinch black pepper

1/8 teaspoon salt

1 cup shredded cheddar cheese (reduced-fat)

Directions

Program the oven temperature to 350°F.

Slice the squash in half and remove the seeds. Arrange the squash, cut side down, in a dish and microwave on high for 20 minutes.

Brown the turkey in a skillet and add the onion and celery. Saute two to three minutes. Blend in the mushrooms, and add the sauce and seasonings. Divide into quarters and spoon into the squash.

Cover and bake for 15 minutes.

Garnish with the cheese and bake until the cheese has melted.

Spicy Sweet Potato Fries

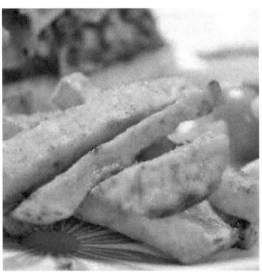

Serves: 4

Time: 40 minutes

Ingredients

1 ½ tablespoons olive oil

2 medium sweet potatoes

¼ teaspoon salt

1 teaspoon ground cumin

½ teaspoon each:

Onion powder

Chili powder

Directions

Program the oven setting to 450°F.

Wash and cut the potatoes lengthwise into fry strips. Combine all ingredients together in a dish and shake

Arrange them on a baking sheet on some parchment paper or foil.

Bake and turn every 5 to 6 minutes - for a total of 20 minutes cooking time.

Spinach Lasagna

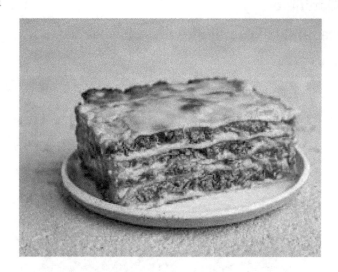

Serves: 8

Time: 2 hours

Ingredients

1 large egg

2 cups cottage cheese (1% milkfat)

2 cups part-skim mozzarella cheese

10 ounces baby spinach

1 jar spaghetti/marinara tomato sauce

1 cup water

9 lasagna noodles

1/8 teaspoon black pepper

Directions

Program the oven temperature to 350°F.

Combine the thawed, drained spinach, one cup of mozzarella, cottage cheese, egg, and the seasonings in a large mixing bowl.

Spray a 9x13x2-inch casserole dish with some cooking spray.

Layer ½ cup of the sauce, 3 noodles, and ½ of the cheese mixture. Repeat, and top with the noodles one cup of mozzarella. Pour water around the edges and toothpicks on top to place a piece of foil over the noodles.

Bake covered for one hour to 1 ½ hours. Let it rest 15 minutes.

Squash and Apple Bake

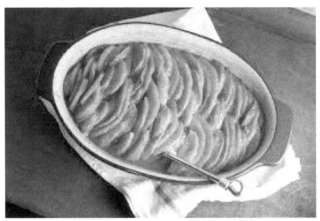

Serves: 6

Time: 70 minutes

Ingredients

2 medium apples

1 medium butternut squash

1 tablespoon each:

Splenda

All-purpose flour

½ teaspoon salt

¼ cup melted butter

2 teaspoons ground cinnamon

Directions

Program the oven temperature to 350°F.

Peel and core the apples and cut them into thin wedges. Peel and cut the squash into ¾-inch cubes.

Combine the squash and apples together in a baking dish.

Add the remainder of ingredients together and add to the top of the mixed apples and squash.

Bake for 50 to 60 minutes in a covered dish. For the last ten minutes, you can remove the top if you prefer the topping crispier.

Eggplant Pesto Mini Pizza

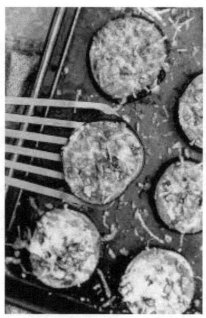

Serves: 4

Time: 55 minutes

Ingredients

1 each chopped:

Bell pepper

Tomato

Eggplant

1 medium sliced red onion

1/8 teaspoon salt

3 cloves of garlic

Pinch of oregano

¼ cup each:

Extra-virgin olive oil

Pesto sauce

Hummus

Vegan Parmesan cheese

Sandwich thins – Arnold Orowheat used

Optional: Pepper flakes

Directions

Set the oven to 400°F.

Chop the vegetables and combine the oil, pepper, salt, oregano, and pepper flakes if desired. Arrange on a baking tin and toast for approximately 30 to 45 minutes or until they are done the way you like them.

Toast the buns and spread the hummus on them, add the veggies, and a bit of pesto sauce. Sprinkle with the vegan cheese and enjoy.

Vegetarian Chili

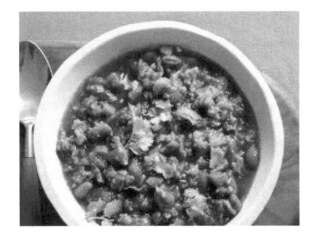

Serves: 8

Time: 15 minutes

Ingredients

1 can (15 ounces) each:

Dark red kidney beans

Pinto beans

Light red kidney beans

Black beans

2 cans (28 ounces) crushed tomatoes

1 can (28 ounces) diced tomatoes

3 cups celery

1 small diced each of bell peppers:

Yellow

 Red

1 medium red onion

4 tablespoons chili powder

3 tablespoons garlic powder

2 tablespoons ground cumin

Directions

Drain and rinse all of the beans. Dice the veggies.

Lightly spray a large pan on the stovetop using medium heat and cook the veggies about six to seven minutes or until they are softened.

Combine the spices, beans, and tomatoes in a slow cooker or a Dutch oven.

Chapter 5: Fruit Salads

California Roll in a Bowl

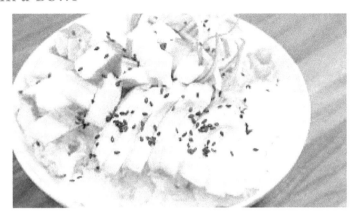

Serves: 4

Time: 15 minutes

Ingredients

1 head chopped lettuce

1 cup cooked brown rice

1 English cucumber – seedless – thinly sliced

1 (8 ounces) package cooked shrimp/crabmeat – chopped

1 grated carrot

1 ripe diced avocado

3 tablespoons pickled ginger

Ingredients for the Dressing

1 tablespoon light soy sauce

½ teaspoon wasabi powder – to taste

3 tablespoons rice wine vinegar

Garnishes:

1 large sheet seaweed/nori (toasted and in small bits)

1 tablespoon sesame seeds

Directions

Combine each of the fixings for the dressing in a mixing dish and whisk well.

Divide it into four sections and enjoy.

Note: You can locate the ginger in the Asian section of the supermarket.

Israeli Salad

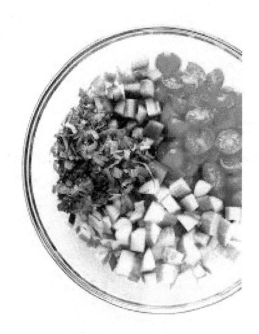

Serves: 8

Time: 5 minutes

Ingredients

1 medium peeled cucumber

3 medium tomatoes

1 yellow/green bell pepper

2 tbsp. lemon juice

3 tbsp. extra-virgin olive oil

1 tsp. of salt and fresh ground pepper

Directions

Chop all of the veggies into small bits.

Combine the rest of the ingredients and enjoy.

Grape Salad

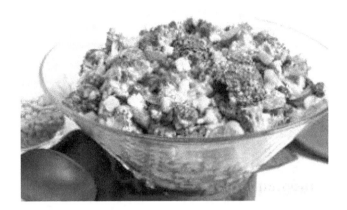

Serves: 16

Time: 65 minutes

Ingredients

2-4 pounds of grapes (green, red, or both)

1 package of fat-free– 8 ounces each:

Sour cream

Softened cream cheese

½ cup each:

Splenda/your choice

Walnuts/Pecans

¼ cup brown sugar

4 tablespoons vanilla extract

Directions

Wash and drain the grapes.

Combine the sour cream, cream cheese, vanilla, and sugar — blending well for about three to four minutes on high with a mixer.

Toss in the grapes and toss until covered.

Pour into a 9x13 cake pan. Sprinkle lightly with the brown sugar. Add the nuts.

Chill about one hour before serving.

Caramel Apple Salad

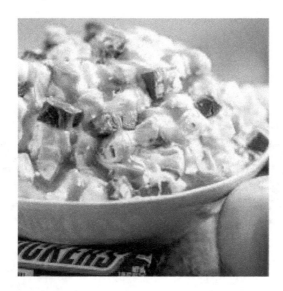

Serves: 16

Time: 30 minutes

Ingredients

1 tub (8 ounces) Cool Whip Free

1 box Instant Butter Scotch Pudding mix (sugar-free)

1 can (14 ounces) pineapple tidbits with the juice

4 large each:

Fuji apples/Red Delicious

Granny Smith apples

Directions

Mix the pineapple with its juice and the pudding mix in a large mixing container.

Dice the apples into small portions and fold in the Cool Whip.

Mix well, and chill in the refrigerator until ready to eat.

Caprese Salad

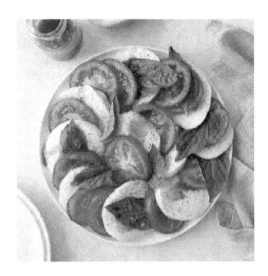

Serves: 2

Time: 10 minutes

Ingredients

6 ounces strawberries

1 ripe avocado

1 (7 ounces) sliced mozzarella ball

Small handful salad leaves

2-3 tablespoons balsamic dressing – your choice

Pepper and salt

Directions

Toss in the salad leaves, avocado, strawberries, and cheese into a serving dish.

Add the tasty dressing and sprinkle with the pepper and salt. Gently toss and enjoy.

Sunshine Fruit Salad

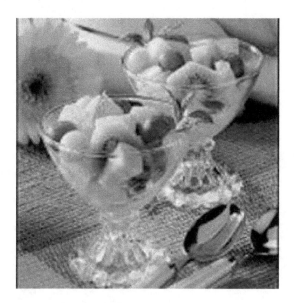

Serves: 10

Time: 65 minutes

Ingredients

2 cans (15 ounces each) mandarin oranges in light syrup

3 cans (20 ounces each) pineapple chunks in 100% juice

2 large bananas

3 medium kiwi fruits – bite-sized

Directions

Drain the oranges and pineapple. Reserve the pineapple juice.

Combine all of the fruit (omit the bananas).

Submerge the fruit with the juice and chill for a minimum of one hour.

Slice and stir in the bananas before serving.

Chapter 6: Snacks and Desserts

Mini Cheesecakes

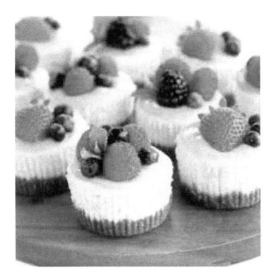

Serves: 20

Time: 2 hours 15 minutes

Ingredients

3 ounces cream cheese

12 ounces fat-free cream cheese

12 low-fat vanilla wafers

½ teaspoon vanilla

½ cup sugar

2 eggs

Cherry pie filling

Directions

Set the oven temperature to 350°F.

Let the cream cheese sit out at room temperature.

Line 12 muffin tins with foil cake liners and add a wafer to each one.

Combine the regular and fat-free cheese until smooth. Blend in the sugar, vanilla, and eggs – beating until smooth.

Pour the batter into the tins and bake for 20 minutes.

Refrigerate for a minimum of two hours – preferably overnight.

Add the cherry filling to each one and serve.

Black Bean Brownies

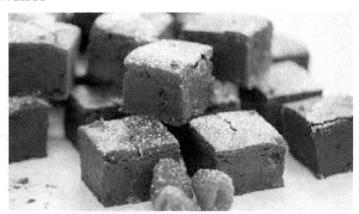

Serves: 16

Time: 40 minutes

Ingredients

4 large eggs

1 can (15 ounces) black beans

3 tablespoons cocoa powder

½ cup granulated Splenda

1 tablespoon instant coffee*

2 tablespoons olive/canola oil

1 teaspoon each:

Baking powder

Vanilla

Directions

Set the oven temperature to 350ºF. Spray an 8x8 pan with some non-stick cooking spray.

*Dissolve the coffee in one tablespoon of hot water and mix with the rest of the ingredients. Drain and rinse the black beans, adding them last.

Bake 30 minutes, and perform the toothpick test for doneness.

Let cool before slicing into 2x2-inch brownies.

Coconut Meringue Cookies

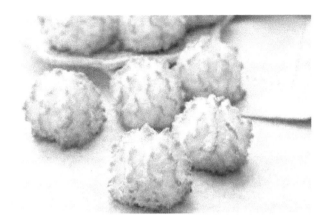

Serves: 20

Time: 30 minutes

Ingredients

2 egg whites

Dash of salt

1 ½ cups coconut sweetened shredded

2/3 cup granulated sugar

¼ teaspoon vanilla extract

Directions

Whip the eggs with a dash of salt to form stiff peaks. Stir in the sugar and fold in the coconut.

Bake 18 to20 minutes at 325ºF.

Healthy Breakfast Cookie

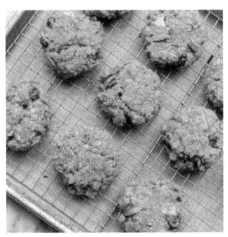

Serves: 30

Time: 20 minutes

Ingredients

2 large eggs

¼ cup butter

½ cup each:

Honey

Chopped - dried apricots

Raisins

1 cup each:

Grated carrots

Chopped walnuts

All-purpose flour

Rolled oats

1 ½ cups Cheerios

1 teaspoon each:

Cinnamon

Nutmeg

Directions

Mix the butter, honey, and egg in a mixing bowl. Combine the mixture with the apricots, walnuts, and raisins.

In a separate container, mix the cinnamon, nutmeg, flour, and oats.

Combine all components and mix well. Fold in the Cheerios.

Drop the dough onto a baking sheet about one inch apart.

Bake 15 minutes or until the cookie is firm.

Blueberry Muffin

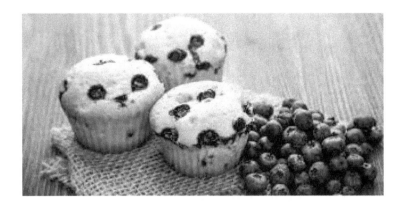

Serves: 12

Time: 35 minutes

Ingredients

1 cup of each:

Flour

Old-fashioned oats

1 tsp. each:

Cinnamon

Baking soda

½ tsp. of salt

½ cup each:

Unsweetened applesauce

Water

Sugar

2 egg whites

1 cup frozen blueberries

Directions

Prepare 12 muffin tins and program the oven to 350°F.

Combine the salt, soda, cinnamon, oats, and flour.

Add the egg whites, sugar, water, and applesauce.

Blend in the blueberries

Bake 20 to 25 minutes until lightly browned.

Pumpkin Muffins

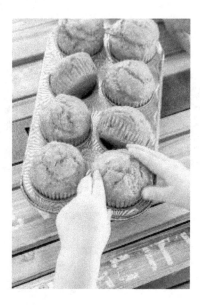

Serves: 18

Time: 40 minutes

Ingredients

1 can/1 pound pumpkin

½ cup flaxseed meal

1 box spice cake mix

Directions

Program the oven to 350°F.

Line a muffin tin with paper liners or cooking spray.

Combine all of the ingredients and bake 25 minutes.

Check for doneness with a toothpick in the center. If it comes out clean – it's done.

Enjoy when you just don't have time for the 'from scratch' recipe.

Conclusion

All bariatric surgeries can have some potential risks and side effects, and as we have already briefly discussed, gastric sleeve surgery is no exception. However, in comparison to other forms of bariatric surgery, gastric sleeve is by far more safe. It's one of the reasons why it's rapidly becoming one of the more popular weight loss surgeries.

In order to give you the most well rounded view of gastric sleeve surgery possible, we'll discuss the possible risks and side effects here.

Moderate Side Effects

-       Moderate side effects can be expected to happen in the days immediately following surgery, but these also go away very quickly and are not dangerous at all. Examples of moderate side effects include pain, bleeding, and swelling.

Severe Side Effects

-       Severe side effects are far less common for gastric sleeve surgery. Some potential complications include stomach acid leaking, inflammation in the stomach, or even bloating in the abdomen. Longer term severe side effects would include infections and pneumonia.

-       While it is a severe side effects, blood clots are extremely rare in patients who undergo gastric sleeve surgery. In fact, less than one percent of all gastric sleeve patients will ever develop blood clots.

-       Remember to take these potential side effects into consideration when you consider any type of bariatric surgery. Also remember that no two patients will ever experience the same combination or same level of risks at the same time. Next, we'll discuss some long term risks of the aftermath of gastric sleeve surgery that can possibly happen overtime.

Risks

-       The first risk that you can take with gastric sleeve surgery is possibly having an allergic reaction to the anesthesia or other medication.

-       Most of the other risks of gastric sleeve surgery would happen in the aftermath, mainly during the two week long recovery period. Examples can include developing infections in the incision area or in the bladder and kidneys, suffer from blood loss, damage to the intestines or organs in the stomach area, sutures becoming rejected, or the intestines becoming blocked.

One thing you have to be aware with gastric sleeve surgery risks is that the risks can develop over the course of several months following the surgery. The good news is that most of these risks can be prevented by simply following your surgeon's Directions, following your dieting regimen, and getting the necessary exercise.

The greatest possible risk of gastric sleeve surgery would be the stomach expanding. If you eat too much food, it can cause your stomach to expand and increase capacity. Remember that your stomach has been reduced by as much as eighty percent, so expanding your stomach beyond the twenty percent it would be after surgery can lead to some potential complications, such as developing malnutrition, lower vitamin levels, kidney stones, or gastritis.

All in all though, don't let these potential risks and side effects dishearten you from undergoing gastric sleeve surgery at all. The chance of you developing any of these risks during or following surgery are very minimal if you follow your doctor's Directions, and gastric sleeve surgery is regarded overall as being one of the safest weight loss surgeries available.

Last but not least, we'll discuss the new diet you'll have to embark on before and after surgery.

Dieting Before Surgery

-       Your stomach and liver are located very closely to one another. When the surgeon will get to your stomach to perform the surgery, they will need to retract your liver with a device to move it out of the way. The overwhelming majority of individuals who are obese will also have fatty liver disease, which is where fat cells will gather around the liver cells, and causes it to function improperly...not to mention increasing the size of it.

-       When the liver expands, it makes it much more difficult for the surgeon to get out of the way, which in turn makes it significantly more difficult for the actual operation and can lead to complications. Therefore, the goal of your diet before gastric sleeve surgery should be to lower the size of the liver via your diet as much as possible.

-       As a large liver will only increase your surgical risk, embarking on a healthy diet before surgery is very important to ensure that the operation proceeds as smoothly as it should. You'd be surprised to know that your liver will decrease in size very quickly if you can adhere to a strict diet in just two weeks before the date of the surgery.

-       Your doctor may recommend a different two week diet than the one we're going to discuss here, but this diet should serve as a golden rule (if you will call it that) for all pre-weight loss surgery diets. Begin by increasing your protein consumption by eating more lean meats, and lower your carbohydrate consumption. This means avoiding bread, pasta and rice. Finally, you'll need to eliminate all sugary foods completely. Candy, juice, soda, cake, you name it.

-       For breakfast, try consuming more protein shakes such as from a supplement store. The only thing to watch out for in these shakes is to make sure that there are no sugars in them. For lunch and dinner alike, focus on eating more vegetables and lean meats.

-       You can eat snacks throughout the day, but only ones that are healthy and low in carbs. Examples of this clued veggies, berries, nuts, and salads. It's also important that you stay hydrated throughout the days, so drinking plenty of water is critically important. An added benefit of water is that it will control the hunger you feel. Plus, it's common knowledge that water is good for you.

- In the three days before surgery, you will have to adhere to a strict liquid diet and stop drinking all beverages that are carbonated and/or have caffeine in them. Clear liquids that you can drink include protein shakes (though less shakes than you were consuming before), water, popsicles (provided they are sugar free), Jell-O, and broth.

- All in all, if you can adhere to this kind of strict surgery, the size of your liver should drastically decrease in the weeks before your surgery and the risk of developing any potential complications during surgery will dramatically decrease.

Dieting After Surgery

- At this point, you have completed the surgery and you may already be home following your stay in the hospital. However, now is no time to return to your previous eating habits. Whereas the previous diet you embarked on was designed to prevent complications from happening during your surgery by reducing the size of your liver, the new diet that you will embark on is focused on preventing the risk of complications after the surgery.

At times, this new diet may seem far more extreme than the previous diet, and even if you find yourself second guessing your decision to have gastric sleeve surgery, just know that this diet is essential to bringing your weight down and preventing the onset of risks. We'll go over what specific foods you can and cannot have for the weeks following your surgery and then beyond that.

- For the first week, you'll have to adhere to clear liquids only. Whereas before you spent two to three days with only clear liquids, you're now going to have to add seven days to that. Fortunately, the ghrelin hormone will be nearly eliminated at this point, so your desire to eat high amounts of 'normal foods' will be nearly eliminated as well. Foods you can eat during this time, provided they are all sugar free, include water, un-carbonated drinks, broth, decaf tea and coffee, jell-o, and popsicles. Specific foods that you should avoid include carbonated drinks, sweet drinks, non-decaf caffeine, and sugar.

- For the second week after surgery, you'll still have to adhere a liquid diet, but with less limitations than the clear liquid diet. For this week, you'll want to add more proteins to the mix. Examples of foods that you can eat during this time include protein powders mixed with liquid, sugar free ice cream, oatmeal, sugarless juices, creamy soups, non fat yogurts, soupy noodles, and sugar free pudding. While this diet definitely has less limitations than before, you can't get too overconfident at this point and eat foods you shouldn't be eating.

- Good news! For the third week after surgery, you'll be able to add some real foods to your diet instead of strictly liquids. However, you should still keep your intake of fats and sugars down if not avoiding them completely. For this week, focus on taking smaller bites and eating the individual bites more slowly, only trying one new food per meal (meaning you should not have two or more kinds of foods at the same meal), and continue to get plenty of protein. This is because you must give your body the time it needs to react to these 'new' foods; remember that's gone well over a month by now without the foods it is used to in taking and digesting. It will need more time to adjust fully.

- There are specific new foods that you can now add to your diet, as well as a few others that you should continue to avoid. New foods that you can add are protein shakes mixed with yogurt and non-fat milk, hummus, low fat cheese, mashed fruit, canned tuna or salmon, mayonnaise, steamed fish (as long as you chew well), scrambled eggs, soup, grounded beef, grounded chicken, soft cereals (tip: allow your cereal to sit in the milk to become soft), soft vegetables, soft cheese, almond milk, and coconut milk. None of these foods should be crunchy and you should remember to chew slowly with all of them.

Foods that you should continue to avoid in the third week are sugars, pasta, rice, bread, fibrous vegetables, and smoothies with high sugar levels.

- For the fourth week, you can continue to introduce more real foods that you're accustomed to. Remember though, your stomach is still very sensitive, and you aren't yet at the point where you can eat anything you want however you want. You still have to eat slowly, eat soft foods whenever possible, and only introduce one new food per meal.

During this time, you should continue consuming protein shakes, as they are one of your best sources of protein throughout this dieting process. You can introduce more fish, fruits, softened vegetables, chicken and beef. All of these foods should be as softened as much as possible and chewed thoroughly. You can also re-introduce potatoes to your diet (mashed, baked and sweetened alike) and cereal. You can also re-introduced caffeine products to your diet, but not to the point that it becomes a regular part of your diet. Be very discretionary as you add caffeine to your diet.

For the fourth week, you should focus primarily on eating three small meals throughout the day and getting plenty of water. But as long as your surgeon approves it, you should also be able to add snacks to your diet at this point. Examples of snacks that you can add include fresh fruit, small portions of baked or sweetened potatoes, small portions of oatmeal, one egg, a small portion of baby carrots, or a small portion of crackers.

Some foods you will have to continue to avoid. Most sodas, fried food, fibrous vegetables, candy and sugar, desserts, pasta, pizzas, whole milk, dairy in general, and nuts will all have to continue to be avoided in the fourth week of your diet.

- For the fifth week, your body will be able to tolerate more foods, but you could still feel an upset stomach at times. Continue to eat three small meals and remain fully hydrated throughout the day. Continue to take your prescribed medication and vitamins, and focus mainly on getting enough protein into your system (sixty grams at the least). Again, protein shakes are an excellent way to get plenty of protein in your system. You should also try to exercise more now, and your body should start to lose weight at a faster rate. Continue to adhere to a strict dieting plan, and when you do eat snacks, only eat from small portions

The Complete Air Fryer Cookbook with Pictures

70+ Perfectly Portioned Air Fryer Recipes for Busy People on a Budget

By

Chef Mirco Miccio

Table of Contents

INTRODUCTION:

The aim of this cookbook is to provide the easiness for those who are professional or doing job somewhere. But with earning, it is also quite necessary to cook food easily & timely instead of ordering hygienic or costly junk food. As we know, after doing office work, no one can cook food with the great effort. For the ease of such people, there are a lot of latest advancements in kitchen accessories. The most popular kitchen appliances usually helps to make foods or dishes like chicken, mutton, beef, potato chips and many other items in less time and budget. There are a lot of things that should be considered when baking with an air fryer. One of the most important tips is to make sure you have all of your equipment ready for the bake. It is best to be prepared ahead of time and this includes having pans, utensils, baking bags, the air fryer itself, and the recipe book instead of using stove or oven. With the help of an air fryer, you can make various dishes for a single person as well as the entire family timely and effortlessly. As there is a famous proverb that "Nothing can be done on its own", it indicates that every task takes time for completion. Some tasks take more time and effort and some requires less time and effort for their completion. Therefore, with the huge range of advancements that come to us are just for our ease. By using appliances like an air fryer comes for the comfort of professional people who are busy in earning their livelihood. In this book, you can follow the latest, delicious, and quick, about 70 recipes that will save your time and provide you healthy food without any great effort.

Chapter # 1:
An Overview & Benefits of an Air Fryer

Introduction:

The most popular kitchen appliance that usually helps to make foods or dishes like chicken, mutton, beef, potato chips and many other items in less time and budget.

Today, everything is materialistic, every person is busy to earn great livelihood. Due to a huge burden of responsibilities, they have no time to cook food on stove after doing hard work. Because, traditionally cooking food on the stove takes more time and effort. Therefore, there are a vast variety of Kitchen appliances. The kitchen appliances are so much helpful in making or cooking food in few minutes and in less budget. You come to home from job, and got too much tired. So, you can cook delicious food in an Air Fryer efficiently and timely as compared to stove. You can really enjoy the food without great effort and getting so much tired.

The Air Fryer Usability:

Be prepared to explore all about frying foods that you learned. To crisp, golden brown excellence (yes, French-fried potatoes and potato chips!), air fryers will fry your favourite foods using minimum or no oil. You can not only make commonly fried foods such as chips and French fries of potatoes, however it is also ideal for proteins, vegetables such as drummettes and chicken wings, coquettes & feta triangles as well as appetizers. And cookies are perfectly cooked in an air fryer, such as brownies and blondies.

The Air Fryer Works as:

- Around 350-375°F (176-190°C) is the ideal temperature of an Air Fryer
- To cook the surface of the food, pour over a food oil at the temperature mentioned above. The oil can't penetrate because it forms a type of seal.
- Simultaneously, the humidity within the food turns into steam that helps to actually cook the food from the inside. It is cleared that the steam helps to maintain the oil out of the food.
- The oil flows into the food at a low temperature, rendering it greasy.
- It oxidizes the oil and, at high temperatures, food will dry out.

On the other hand, an air fryer is similar to a convection oven, but in a diverse outfit, food preparation done at very high temperatures whereas, inside it, dry air circulates around the food at the same time, while making it crisp without putting additional fat, it makes it possible for cooking food faster.

What necessary to Search for in an Air Fryer?

As we know, several different sizes and models of air fryers are available now. If you're cooking for a gathering, try the extra-large air fryer, that can prepare or fry a whole chicken, other steaks or six servings of French fries.

Suppose, you've a fixed counter space, try the Large Air Fryer that uses patented machinery to circulate hot air for sufficient, crispy results. The latest air fryer offers an extra compact size with identical capacity! and tar equipment, which ensures that food is cooking evenly (no further worries of build-ups). You will be able to try all the fried foods you enjoy, with no embarrassment.

To increase the functionality of an air fryer, much more, you can also purchase a wide range of different accessories, including a stand, roasting pan, muffin cups, and mesh baskets. Check out the ingredients of our air fryer we created, starting from buttermilk with black pepper seasoning to fry chicken or Sichuan garlic seasoning suitable for Chinese cuisine.

We will read about the deep fryer, with tips and our favourite recipes like burgers, chicken wings, and many more.

Most Common - Five Guidelines for an Air Fryer usage:

1. Shake the food.

Open the air fryer and shake the foods efficiently because the food is to "fry" in the machine's basket—Light dishes like Sweet French fries and Garlic chips will compress. Give Rotation to the food every 5-10 mins for better performance

2. Do not overload.

Leave enough space for the food so that the air circulates efficiently; so that's gives you crunchy effects. Our kitchen testing cooks trust that the snacks and small batches can fry in air fryer.

3. Slightly spray to food.

Gently spray on food by a cooking spray bottle and apply a touch of oil on food to make sure the food doesn't stick to the basket.

4. Retain an Air fry dry.

Beat food to dry before start cooking (even when marinated, e.g.) to prevent splashing & excessive smoke. Likewise, preparing high-fat foods such as chicken steaks or wings, be assured to remove the grease from the lower part of machine regularly.

5. Other Most Dominant cooking techniques.

The air fryer is not just for deep frying; It is also perfect for further safe methods of cooking like baking, grilling, roasting and many more. Our kitchen testing really loves using the unit for cooking salmon in air fryer!

An Air Fryer Helps to reduce fat content

Generally, food cooked in deep fryer contains higher fat level than preparing food in other cooking appliances. For Example; a fried chicken breast contains about 30% more fat just like a fat level in roasted chicken

Many Manufacturers claimed, an Air fryer can reduce fat from fried food items up-to 75%. So, an air fryer requires less amount of fat than a deep fryer. As, many dishes cooked in deep fryer consume 75% oil (equal to 3 cups) and an air fryer prepare food by applying the oil in just about 1 tablespoon (equal to 15ml).

One research tested the potato chips prepared in air fryer characteristics then observed: the air frying method produces a final product with slightly lower fat but same moisture content and color. So, there is a major impact on anyone's health, an excessive risk of illnesses such as inflammation, infection and heart disease has been linked to a greater fat intake from vegetable oils.

Air Fryer provides an Aid in Weight Loss

The dishes prepared deep fryer are not just having much fat but also more in calories that causes severe increase in weight. Another research of 33,542 Spanish grown-ups indicates that a greater usage of fried food linked with a higher occurrence of obesity. Dietetic fat has about twice like many calories per gram while other macro-nutrients such as carbohydrates, vitamins and proteins, averaging in at 9 calories throughout each and every gram of oil or fat.

By substituting to air fryer is an easy way to endorse in losing weight and to reduce calories and it will be done only by taking food prepared in air fryer.

Air Fried food may reduce the potentially harmful chemicals

Frying foods can produce potentially hazardous compounds such as acrylamide, in contrast to being higher in fat and calories. An acrylamide is a compound that is formed in carbohydrate- rich dishes or foods during highly-heated cooking methods such as frying. Acrylamide is known as a "probable carcinogen" which indicates as some research suggests that it could be associated with the development of cancer. Although the findings are conflicting, the link between dietary acrylamide and a greater risk of kidney, endometrial and ovarian cancers has been identified in some reports. Instead of cooking food in a deep fryer, air frying your food may aid the acrylamide content. Some researches indicates that air-frying method may cut the acrylamide by 90% by comparing deep frying method. All other extremely harmful chemicals produced by high-heat cooking are polycyclic aromatic hydrocarbons, heterocyclic amines and aldehydes and may be associated with a greater risk of cancer. That's why, the air fried food may help to reduce the chance of extremely dangerous chemicals or compounds and maintain your health.

Chapter # 2:

70 Perfectly Portioned Air Fryer Recipes for Busy People in Minimum Budget

1. Air fried corn, zucchini and haloumi fritters

Ingredients

- Coarsely grated block haloumi - 225g
- Coarsely grated Zucchini - 2 medium sized
- Frozen corn kernels - 150g (1 cup)
- Lightly whisked eggs - 2
- Self-raising flour - 100g
- Extra virgin olive oil - to drizzle
- Freshly chopped oregano leaves - 3 tablespoons
- Fresh oregano extra sprigs - to serve
- Yoghurt - to serve

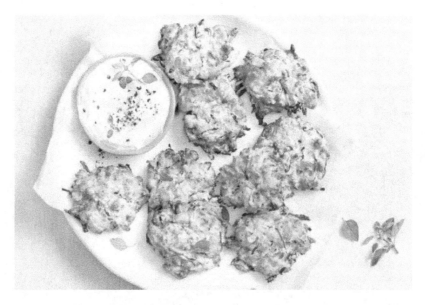

Method

1. Use your palms to squeeze out the extra liquid from the zucchini and place them in a bowl. Add the corn and haloumi and stir for combining them. Then add the eggs, oregano and flour. Add seasoning and stir until fully mixed.
2. Set the temperature of an air fryer to 200 C. Put spoonsful of the mixture of zucchini on an air fryer. Cook until golden and crisp, for 8 minutes. Transfer to a dish that is clean. Again repeat this step by adding the remaining mixture in 2 more batches.

3. Take a serving plate and arrange soft fritters on it. Take yoghurt in a small serving bowl. Add seasoning of black pepper on the top of yoghurt. Drizzle with olive oil. At the end, serve this dish with extra oregano.

2. Air fryer fried rice

Ingredients

- Microwave long grain rice - 450g packet
- Chicken tenderloins - 300g
- Rindless bacons - 4 ranchers
- Light Soy sauce - 2 tablespoons
- Oyster sauce - 2 tablespoons
- Sesame oil - 1 tablespoon
- Fresh finely grated ginger - 3 tablespoons
- Frozen peas - 120g (3/4 cup)
- Lightly whisked eggs - 2
- Sliced green shallots - 2
- Thin sliced red chilli - 1
- Oyster sauce - to drizzle

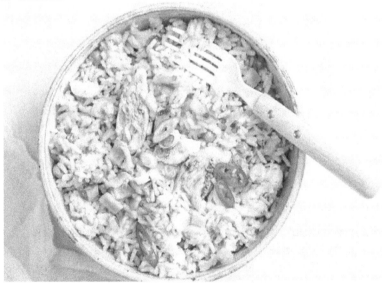

Method
1. Set the 180°C temperature of an air fryer. Bacon and chicken is placed on the rack of an air fryer. Cook them until fully cooked for 8-10 minutes. Shift it to a clean plate and set this plate aside to cool. Then, slice and chop the bacon and chicken.
2. In the meantime, separate the rice grains in the packet by using your fingers. Heat the rice for 60 seconds in a microwave. Shift to a 20cm ovenproof, round high-sided pan or dish. Apply the sesame oil, soy sauce, ginger, oyster sauce and 10ml water and mix well.

3. Put a pan/dish in an air fryer. Cook the rice for 5 minutes till them soft. Then whisk the chicken, half of bacon and peas in the eggs. Completely cook the eggs in 3 minutes. Mix and season the top of half shallot with white pepper and salt.

4. Serve with the seasoning of chilli, remaining bacon and shallot and oyster sauce.

3. Air fried banana muffins

Ingredients
- Ripe bananas - 2
- Brown sugar - 60g (1/3 cup)
- Olive oil - 60ml (1/4 cup)
- Buttermilk - 60ml (1/4 cup)
- Self-raising flour - 150g (1 cup)
- Egg - 1
- Maple syrup - to brush or to serve

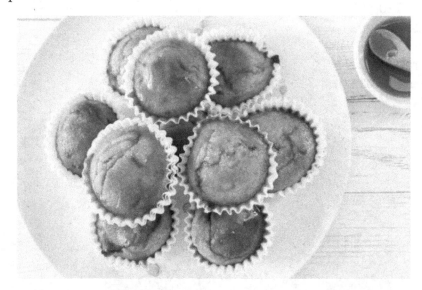

Method
1. Mash the bananas in a small bowl using a fork. Until needed, set aside.

2. In a medium cup, whisk the flour and sugar using a balloon whisk. In the middle, make a well. Add the buttermilk, oil and egg. Break up the egg with the help of a whisk. Stir by using wooden spoon until the mixture is mixed. Stir the banana through it.

3. Set the temperature of an air fryer at 180C. Splits half of the mixture into 9 cases of patties. Remove the rack from the air fryer and pass the cases to the rack carefully. Switch the rack back to the fryer. Bake the muffins completely by cooking them for 10 minutes. Move to the wire rack. Repeat this step on remaining mixture to produce 18 muffins.

4. Brush the muffin tops with maple syrup while they're still warm. Serve, if you like, with extra maple syrup.

4. Air fried Nutella brownies

Ingredients
- Plain flour - 150g (1 cup)
- Castor white sugar - 225g (1 cup)
- Lightly whisked eggs - 3
- Nutella - 300g (1 cup)
- Cocoa powder - to dust

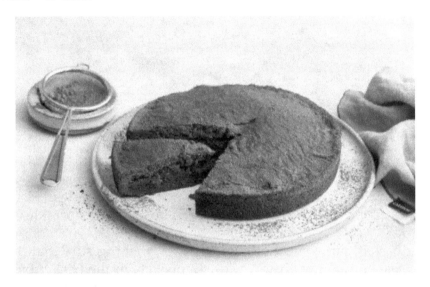

Method
1. Apply butter in a 20cm circular cake pan. Cover the base by using baking paper.
2. Whisk the flour and sugar together in a bowl by using balloon whisk. In the middle, make a well. Add the Nutella and egg in the middle of bowl by making a well. Stir with a large metal spoon until mixed. Move this mixture to the previously prepared pan and smooth the surface of the mixture by using metal spoon.
3. Pre - heat an air fryer to 160C. Bake the brownie about 40 minutes or until a few crumbs stick out of a skewer inserted in the middle. Fully set aside to cool.
4. Garnish the top of the cake by dusting them with cocoa powder, and cut them into pieces. Brownies are ready to be served.

5. Air fried celebration bites

Ingredients
- Frozen shortcrust partially thawed pastry - 4 sheets
- Lightly whisked eggs - 1
- Unrapped Mars Celebration chocolates - 24
- Icing sugar - to dust
- Cinnamon sugar - to dust
- Whipped cream - to serve

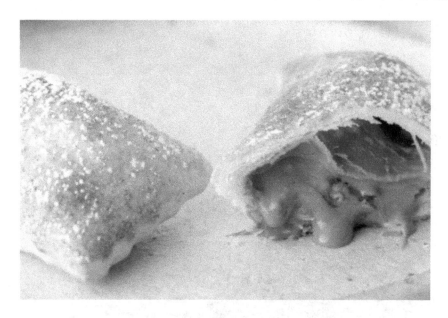

Method

1. Slice each pastry sheet into 6 rectangles. Brush the egg gently. One chocolate is placed in the middle of each rectangular piece of pastry. Fold the pastry over to cover the chocolate completely. Trim the pastry, press and seal the sides. Place it on a tray containing baking paper. Brush the egg on each pastry and sprinkle cinnamon sugar liberally.

2. In the air-fryer basket, put a sheet of baking paper, making sure that the paper is 1 cm smaller than the basket to allow airflow. Put six pockets in the basket by taking care not to overlap. Cook for 8-9 minutes at 190°C until pastries are completely cooked with golden color. Shift to a dish. Free pockets are then used again.

3. Sprinkle Icing sugar on the top of tasty bites. Serve them with a whipped cream to intensify its flavor.

6. Air fried nuts and bolts

Ingredients

- Dried farfalle pasta - 2 cups
- Extra virgin olive oil - 60ml (1/4th cup)
- Brown sugar - 2 tablespoons
- Onion powder - 1 tablespoon
- Smoked paprika - 2 tablespoons
- Chili powder - 1/2 tablespoon
- Garlic powder - 1/2 tablespoon
- Pretzels - 1 cup
- Raw macadamias - 80g (1/2 cup)
- Raw cashews - 80g (1/2 cup)
- Kellog's Nutri-grain cereal - 1 cup
- Sea salt - 1 tablespoon

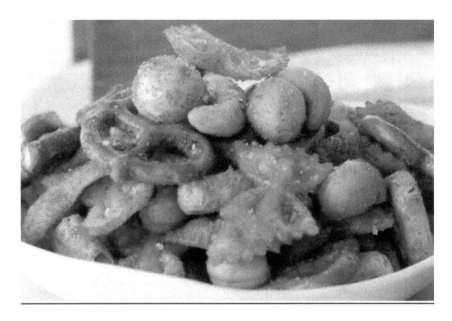

Method

1. Take a big saucepan of boiling salted water, cook the pasta until just ready and soft. Drain thoroughly. Shift pasta to a tray and pat with a paper towel to dry. Move the dried pasta to a wide pot.

2. Mix the sugar, oil, onion, paprika, chili and garlic powders together in a clean bowl. Add half of this mixture in the bowl containing pasta. Toss this bowl slightly for the proper coating of mixture over pasta.

3. Set the temperature at 200C of an Air Fryer. Put the pasta in air fryer's pot. After cooking for 5 minutes, shake the pot and cook for more 5-7 minutes, until they look golden and crispy. Shift to a wide bowl.

4. Take the pretzels in a bowl with the nuts and apply the remaining mixture of spices. Toss this bowl for the proper coating. Put in air fryer's pot and cook at 180C for 3-4 minutes. Shake this pot and cook for more 2-3 minutes until it's golden in color. First add pasta and then add the cereal. Sprinkle salt on it and toss to mix properly. Serve this dish after proper cooling.

7. Air fried coconut shrimps

Ingredients

- Plain flour - 1/2 cup
- Eggs - 2
- Bread crumbs - 1/2 cup
- Black pepper powder - 1.5 teaspoons
- Sweetless flaked coconut - 3/4 cup
- Uncooked, deveined and peeled shrimp - 12 ounces
- Salt - 1/2 teaspoon
- Honey - 1/4 cup
- Lime juice - 1/4 cup
- Finely sliced serrano chili - 1

- Chopped cilantro - 2 teaspoons
- Cooking spray

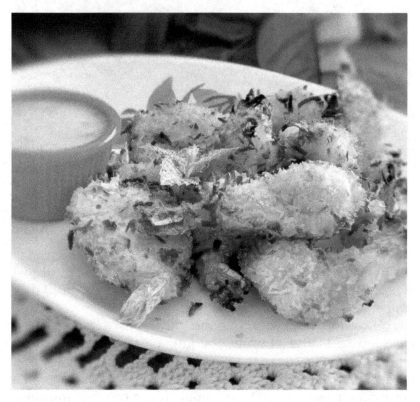

Method

1. Stir the pepper and flour in a clean bowl together. Whisk the eggs in another bowl and h panko and coconut in separate bowl.   Coat the shrimps with flour mixture by holding each shrimp by tail and shake off the extra flour.   Then coat the floured shrimp with egg and allow it to drip off excess. Give them the final coat of coconut mixture and press them to stick. Shift on a clean plate. Spray shrimp with cooking oil.

2. Set the temperature of the air-fryer to 200C. In an air fryer, cook half of the shrimp for 3 minutes. Turn the shrimp and cook further for more 3 minutes until color changes in golden. Use 1/4 teaspoon of salt for seasoning. Repeat this step for the rest of shrimps.

3. In the meantime, prepare a dip by stirring lime juice, serrano chili and honey in a clean bowl.

4. Serve fried shrimps with sprinkled cilantro and dip.

8. Air fried Roasted Sweet and Spicy Carrots

Ingredients

- Cooking oil
- Melted butter - 1 tablespoon
- Grated orange zest - 1 teaspoon

- Carrots - 1/2 pound
- Hot honey - 1 tablespoon
- Cardamom powder - 1/2 teaspoon
- Fresh orange juice - 1 tablespoon
- Black pepper powder - to taste
- Salt - 1 pinch

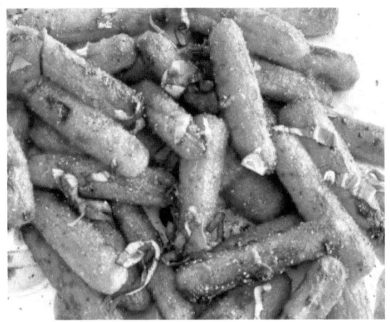

Method

1. Set the temperature of an air to 200C. Lightly coat its pot with cooking oil.

2. Mix honey, cardamom and orange zest in a clean bowl. Take 1 tablespoon of this sauce in another bowl and place aside. Coat carrots completely by tossing them in remaining sauce. Shift carrots to an air fryer pot.

3. Air fry the carrots and toss them after every 6 minutes. Cook carrots for 15-20 minutes until they are fully cooked and roasted. Combine honey butter sauce with orange juice to make sauce. Coat carrots with this sauce. Season with black pepper and salt and serve this delicious dish.

9. Air fried Chicken Thighs

Ingredients

- Boneless chicken thighs - 4
- Extra virgin olive oil - 2 teaspoons
- Smoked paprika - 1 teaspoon
- Salt - 1/2 teaspoon
- Garlic powder - 3/4 teaspoon
- Black pepper powder - 1/2 teaspoon

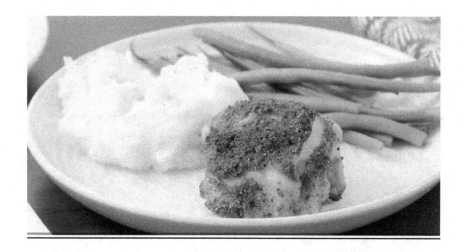

Method

1. Set the temperature of an air fryer to 200C.
2. Dry chicken thighs by using tissue paper. Brush olive oil on the skin side of each chicken thigh. Shift the single layer of chicken thighs on a clean tray.
3. Make a mixture of salt, black pepper, paprika and garlic powder in a clean bowl. Use a half of this mixture for the seasoning of 4 chicken thighs on both sides evenly. Then shift single layer of chicken thighs in an air fryer pot by placing skin side up.
4. Preheat the air fryer and maintain its temperature to 75C. Fry chicken for 15-18 minutes until its water become dry and its color changes to brown. Serve immediately.

10. Air fried French Fries

Ingredients
- Peeled Potatoes - 1 pound
- Vegetable oil - 2 tablespoon
- Cayenne pepper - 1 pinch
- Salt - 1/2 teaspoon

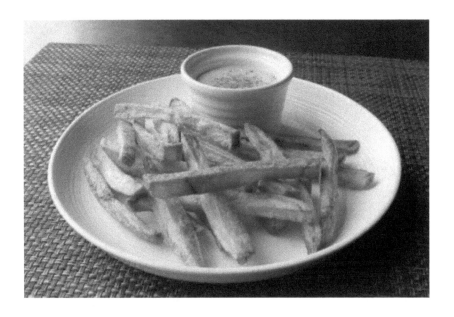

Method
1. Lengthwise cut thick slices of potato of 3/8 inches.
2. Soak sliced potatoes for 5 minutes in water. Drain excess starch water from soaked potatoes after 5 minutes. Place these potatoes in boiling water pan for 8-10 minutes.
3. Remove water from the potatoes and dry them completely. Cool them for 10 minutes and shift in a clean bowl. Add some oil and fully coat the potatoes with cayenne by tossing.
4. Set the temperature of an air fryer to 190C. Place two layers of potatoes in air fryer pot and cook them for 10-15 minutes. Toss fries continuously and cook for more 10 minutes until their color changes to golden brown. Season fries with salt and serve this appetizing dish immediately.

11. Air fried Mini Breakfast Burritos

Ingredients
- Mexican style chorizo - 1/4 cup
- Sliced potatoes - 1/2 cup
- Chopped serrano pepper - 1
- 8-inch flour tortillas - 4
- Bacon grease - 1 tablespoon
- Chopped onion - 2 tablespoon
- Eggs - 2
- Cooking avacado oil - to spray
- Salt - to taste
- Black pepper powder - to taste

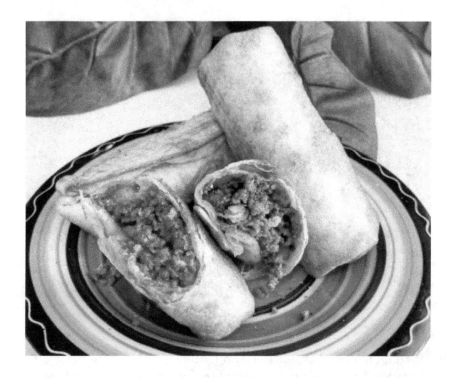

Method

1. Take chorizo in a large size pan and cook on medium flame for 8 minutes with continuous stirring until its color change into reddish brown. Shift chorizo in a clean plate and place separate.

2. Take bacon grease in same pan and melt it on medium flame. Place sliced potatoes and cook them for 10 minutes with constant stirring. Add serrano pepper and onion meanwhile. Cook for more 2-5 minutes until potatoes are fully cooked, onion and serrano pepper become soften. Then add chorizo and eggs and cook for more 5 minutes until potato mixture is fully incorporated. Use pepper and salt for seasoning.

3. In the meantime, heat tortillas in a large pan until they become soft and flexible. Put 1/3 cup of chorizo mixture at the center of each tortilla. Filling is covered by rolling the upper and lower side of tortilla and give shape of burrito. Spray cooking oil and place them in air fryer pot.

4. Fry these burritos at 200C for 5 minutes. Change the side'scontinuously and spray with cooking oil. Cook in air fryer for 3-4 minutes until color turns into light brown. Shift burritos in a clean dish and serve this delicious dish.

12. Air fried Vegan Tator Tots

Ingredients
- Frozen potato nuggets (Tator Tots) - 2 cups
- Buffalo wing sauce - 1/4 cup
- Vegan ranch salad - 1/4 cup

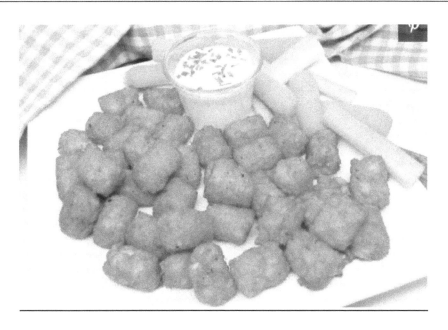

Method

1. Set the temperature of an air fryer to 175C.
2. Put frozen potato nuggets in air fryer pot and cook for 6-8 minutes with constant shake.
3. Shift potatoes to a large-sized bowl and add wing sauce. Combine evenly by tossing them and place them again in air fryer pot.
4. Cook more for 8-10 minutes without disturbance. Shift to a serving plate. Serve with ranch dressing and enjoy this dish.

13. Air fried Roasted Cauliflower

Ingredients
- Cauliflower florets - 4 cups
- Garlic - 3 cloves
- Smoked paprika - 1/2 teaspoon
- Peanut oil - 1 tablespoon
- Salt - 1/2 teaspoon

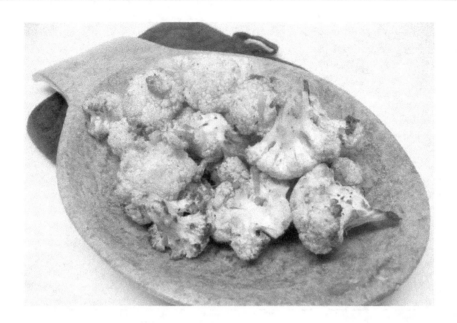

Method
1. Set the temperature of an air fryer to 200C.
2. Smash garlic cloves with a knife and mix with salt, oil and paprika. Coat cauliflower in this mixture.
3. Put coated cauliflower in air fryer pot and cook around 10-15 minutes with stirring after every 5 minutes. Cook according to desired color and crispiness and serve immediately.

14. Air fried Cinnamon-Sugar Doughnuts

Ingredients
- White sugar - 1/2 cup
- Brown sugar - 1/4 cup
- Melted butter - 1/4 cup
- Cinnamon powder - 1 teaspoon
- Ground nutmeg - 1/4 TEASPOON
- Packed chilled flaky biscuit dough - 1 (16.3 ounce)

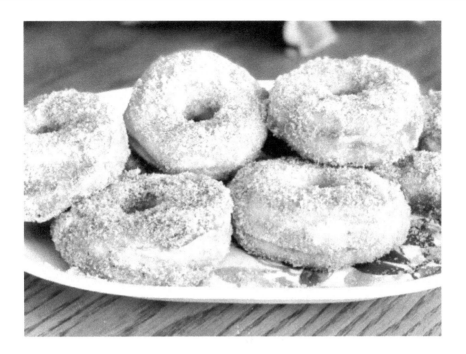

Method
1. Put melted butter in a clean bowl. Add brown sugar, white sugar, nutmeg and cinnamon and mix.
2. Divide and cut biscuit dough into many single biscuits and give them the shape of doughnuts using a biscuit cutter. Shift doughnuts in an air fryer pot.
3. Air fry the doughnuts for 5-6 minutes at 175C until color turns into golden brown. Turn the side of doughnuts and cook for more 1-3 minutes.
4. Shift doughnuts from air fryer to a clean dish and dip them in melted butter. Then completely coat these doughnuts in sugar and cinnamon mixture and serve frequently.

15. Air Fried Broiled Grapefruit

Ingredients
- Chilled red grapefruit - 1
- Melted butter - 1 tablespoon
- Brown sugar - 2 tablespoon
- Ground cinnamon - 1/2 teaspoon
- Aluminium foil

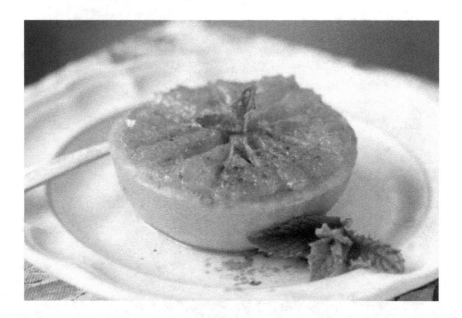

Method

1. Set the temperature of an air fryer to 200C.
2. Cut grapefruit crosswise to half and also cut a thin slice from one end of grapefruit for sitting your fruit flat on a plate.
3. Mix brown sugar in melted butter in a small sized bowl. Coat the cut side of the grapefruit with this mixture. Dust the little brown sugar over it.
4. Take 2 five inch pieces of aluminium foil and put the half grapefruit on each piece. Fold the sides evenly to prevent juice leakage. Place them in air fryer pot.
5. Broil for 5-7 minutes until bubbling of sugar start in an air fryer. Before serving, sprinkle cinnamon on grapefruit.

16. Air Fried Brown Sugar and Pecan Roasted Apples

Ingredients

- Apples - 2 medium
- Chopped pecans - 2 tablespoons
- Plain flour - 1 teaspoon
- Melted butter - 1 tablespoon
- Brown sugar - 1 tablespoon
- Apple pie spice - 1/4 teaspoon

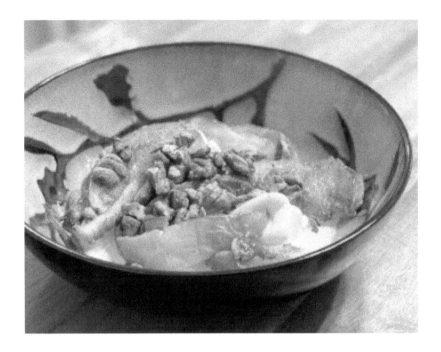

Method

1. Set the temperature of an air fryer to 180C.

2. Mix brown sugar, pecan, apple pie spice and flour in a clean bowl. Cut apples in wedges and put them in another bowl and coat them with melted butter by tossing. Place a single layer in an air fryer pot and add mixture of pecan on the top.

3. Cook apples for 12-15 minutes until they get soft.

17. Air Fried Breaded Sea Scallops

Ingredients

- Crushed butter crackers - 1/2 cup
- Seafood seasoning - 1/2 teaspoon
- Sea scallops - 1 pound
- Garlic powder - 1/2 teaspoon
- Melted butter - 2 tablespoons
- Cooking oil - for spray

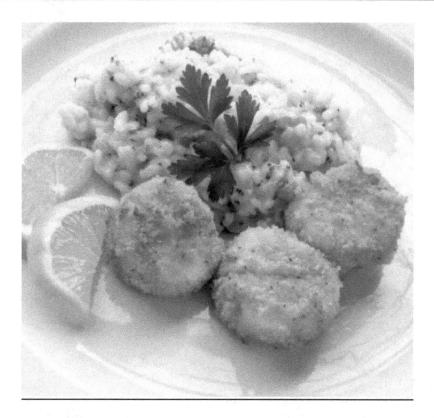

Method

1. Set the temperature of an air fryer to 198C.

2. Combine garlic powder, seafood seasoning and cracker crumbs in a clean bowl. Take melted butter in another bowl.

3. Coat each scallop with melted butter. Then roll them in breading until completely enclose. Place them on a clean plate and repeat this step with rest of the scallops.

4. Slightly spray scallops with cooking oil and place them on the air fryer pot at equal distance. You may work in 2-3 batches.

5. Cook them for 2-3 minutes in preheated air fryer. Use a spatula to change the side of each scallop. Cook for more 2 minutes until they become opaque. Dish out in a clean plate and serve immediately.

18. Air Fried Crumbed Fish

Ingredients

- Flounder fillets - 4
- Dry bread crumbs - 1 cup
- Egg - 1
- Sliced lemon - 1
- Vegetable oil - 1/4 cup

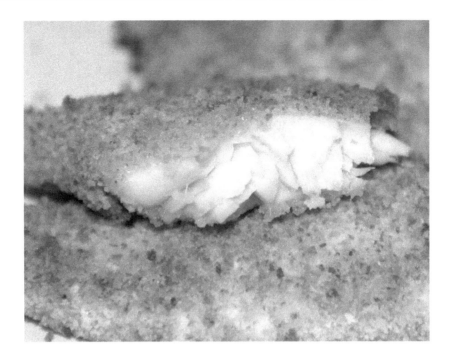

Method
1. Set the temperature of an air fryer to 180C.
2. Combine oil and bread crumbs in a clean bowl and mix them well.
3. Coat each fish fillets with beaten egg, then evenly dip them in the crumbs mixture.
4. Place coated fillets in preheated air fryer and cook for 10-12 minutes until fish easily flakes by touching them with fork. Shift prepared fish in a clean plate and serve with lemon slices.

19. Air Fried Cauliflower and Chickpea Tacos

Ingredients

- Cauliflower - 1 small
- Chickpeas - 15 ounce
- Chili powder - 1 teaspoon
- Cumin powder - 1 teaspoon
- Lemon juice - 1 tablespoon
- Sea salt - 1 teaspoon
- Garlic powder - 1/4 teaspoon
- Olive oil - 1 tablespoon

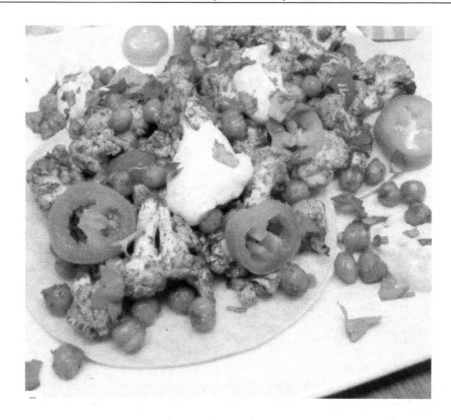

Method

1. Set the temperature of an air fryer to 190C.

2. Mix lime juice, cumin, garlic powder, salt, olive oil and chili powder in a clean bowl. Now coat well the cauliflower and chickpeas in this mixture by constant stirring.

3. Put cauliflower mixture in an air fryer pot. Cook for 8-10 minutes with constant stirring. Cook for more 10 minutes and stir for final time. Cook for more 5 minutes until desired crispy texture is attained.

5. Place cauliflower mixture by using spoon and serve.

20. Air Fried Roasted Salsa

Ingredients

- Roma tomatoes - 4
- Seeded Jalapeno pepper - 1
- Red onion - 1/2
- Garlic - 4 cloves
- Cilantro - 1/2 cup
- Lemon juice - 1
- Cooking oil - to spray

- Salt - to taste

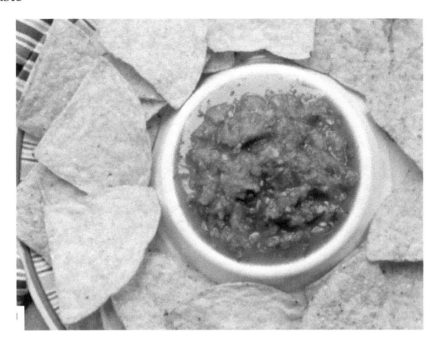

Method

1. Set the temperature of an air fryer to 200C.

2. Put tomatoes, red onion and skin side down of jalapeno in an air fryer pot. Brush lightly these vegetables with cooking oil for roasting them easily.

3. Cook vegetables in an air fryer for 5 minutes. Then add garlic cloves and again spray with cooking oil and fry for more 5 minutes.

4. Shift vegetables to cutting board and allow them to cool for 8-10 minutes.

5. Separate skins of jalapeno and tomatoes and chop them with onion into large pieces. Add them to food processor bowl and add lemon juice, cilantro, garlic and salt. Pulsing for many times until all the vegetables are evenly chopped. Cool them for 10-15 minutes and serve this delicious dish immediately.

21. Air Fried Flour Tortilla Bowls

Ingredients

- Flour tortilla - 1 (8 inch)
- Souffle dish - 1 (4 1/2 inch)

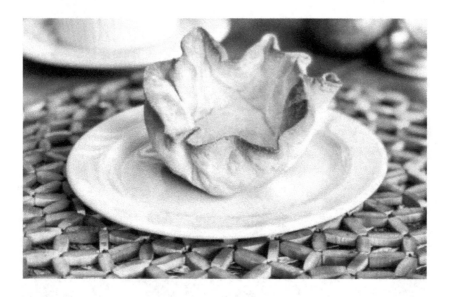

Method

1. Set the temperature of an air fryer to 190C.

2. Take tortilla in a large pan and heat it until it become soft. Put tortilla in the souffle dish by patting down side and fluting up from its sides of dish.

3. Air fry tortilla for 3-5 minutes until its color change into golden brown.

4. Take out tortilla bowl from the dish and put the upper side in the pot. Air fry again for more 2 minutes until its color turns into golden brown. Dish out and serve.

22. Air Fried Cheese and Mini Bean Tacos

Ingredients

- Can Refried beans - 16 ounce
- American cheese - 12 slices
- Flour tortillas - 12 (6 inch)
- Taco seasoning mix - 1 ounce
- Cooking oil - to spray

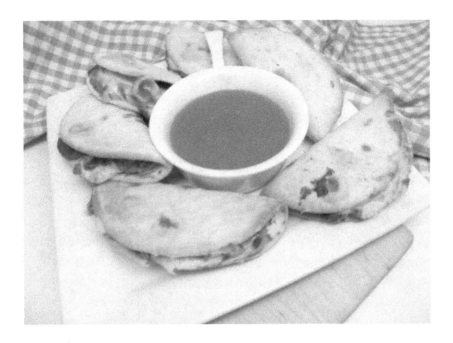

Method

1. Set the temperature of an air fryer to 200C.

2. Combine refried beans and taco seasoning evenly in a clean bowl and stir.

3. Put 1 slice of cheese in the center of tortilla and place 1 tablespoon of bean mixture over cheese. Again place second piece of cheese over this mixture. Fold tortilla properly from upper side and press to enclose completely. Repeat this step for the rest of beans, cheese and tortillas.

4. Spray cooking oil on the both sides of tacos. Put them in an air fryer at equal distance. Cook the tacos for 3 minutes and turn it side and again cook for more 3 minutes. Repeat this step for the rest of tacos. Transfer to a clean plate and serve immediately.

23. Air Fried Lemon Pepper Shrimp

Ingredients

- Lemon - 1
- Lemon pepper - 1 teaspoon
- Olive oil - 1 tablespoon
- Garlic powder - 1/4 teaspoon
- Paprika - 1/4 teaspoon
- Deveined and peeled shrimps - 12 ounces
- Sliced lemon – 1

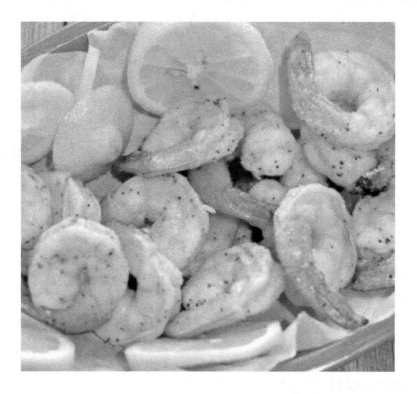

Method

1. Set the temperature of an air fryer to 200C.

2. Mix lemon pepper, garlic powder, and olive oil, paprika and lemon juice in a clean bowl. Coat shrimps by this mixture by tossing.

3. Put shrimps in an air fryer and cook for 5-8 minutes until its color turn to pink. Dish out cooked shrimps and serve with lemon slices.

24. Air Fried Shrimp a la Bang Bang

Ingredients

- Deveined raw shrimps - 1 pound
- Sweet chili sauce - 1/4 cup
- Plain flour - 1/4 cup
- Green onions - 2
- Mayonnaise - 1/2 cup
- Sriracha sauce - 1 tablespoon
- Bread crumbs - 1 cup
- Leaf lettuce - 1 head

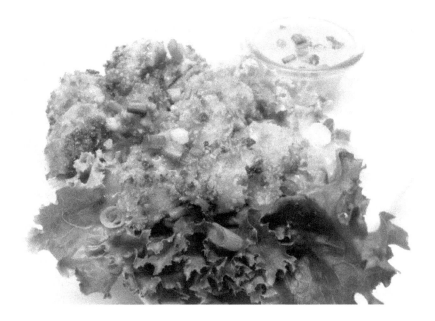

Method

1. Set the temperature of an air fryer to 200C

2. Make a bang bang sauce by mixing chili sauce, mayonnaise and sriracha sauce in a clean bowl. Separate some sauce for dipping in a separate small bowl.

3. Place bread crumbs and flour in two different plates. Coat shrimps with mayonnaise mixture, then with flour and then bread crumbs. Set coated shrimps on a baking paper.

4. Place them in an air fryer pot and cook for 10-12 minutes. Repeat this step for the rest of shrimps. Transfer shrimps to a clean dish and serve with green onions and lettuce.

25. Air Fried Spicy Bay Scallops

Ingredients

- Bay scallops - 1 pound
- Chili powder - 2 teaspoons
- Smoked paprika- 2 teaspoons
- Garlic powder - 1 teaspoon
- Olive oil - 2 teaspoons
- Black pepper powder - 1/4 teaspoon
- Cayenne red pepper - 1/8 teaspoon

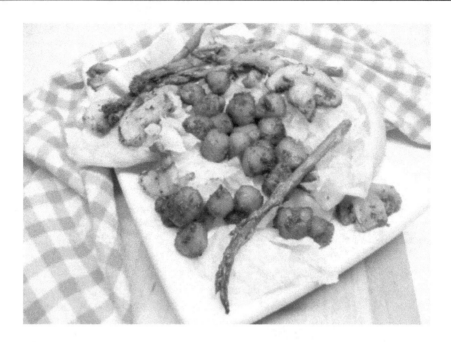

Method

1. Set the temperature of an air fryer to 200C

2. Mix smoked paprika, olive oil, bay scallops, garlic powder, pepper, chili powder and cayenne pepper in a clean bowl and stir properly. Shift this mixture to an air fryer.

3. Air fry for 6-8 minutes with constant shaking until scallops are fully cooked. Transfer this dish in a clean plate and serve immediately.

26. Air Fried Breakfast Fritatta

Ingredients

- Fully cooked breakfast sausages - 1/4 pound
- Cheddar Monterey Jack cheese - 1/2 cup
- Green onion - 1
- Cayenne pepper - 1 pinch
- Red bell pepper - 2 tablespoons
- Eggs - 4
- Cooking oil - to spray

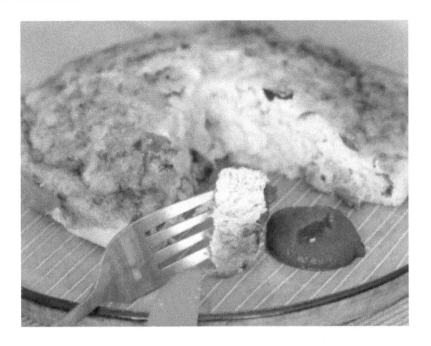

Method

1. Set the temperature of an air fryer to 180C.

2. Mix eggs, sausages, Cheddar Monterey Jack cheese, onion, bell pepper and cayenne in a clean bowl and stir to mix properly.

3. Spray cooking oil on a clean non-stick cake pan. Put egg mixture in the cake pan. Air fry for 15-20 minutes until fritatta is fully cooked and set. Transfer it in a clean plate and serve immediately.

27. Air Fried Roasted Okra

Ingredients

- Trimmed and sliced Okra - 1/2 pound
- Black pepper powder - 1/8 teaspoon
- Olive oil - 1 teaspoon
- Salt - 1/4 teaspoon

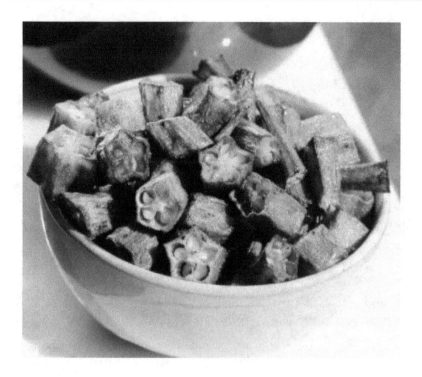

Method

1. Set the temperature of an air fryer to 175C.

2. Mix olive oil, black pepper, salt and okra in a clean bowl and stir to mix properly.

3. Make a single layer of this mixture in an air fryer pot. Air fry for 5-8 minutes with constant stirring. Cook for more 5 minutes and again toss. Cook for more 3 minutes and dish out in a clean plate and serve immediately.

28. Air Fried Rib-Eye Steak

Ingredients

- Rib-eye steak - 2 (1 1/2 inch thick)
- Olive oil - 1/4 cup
- Grill seasoning - 4 teaspoons
- Reduced sodium soy sauce - 1/2 cup

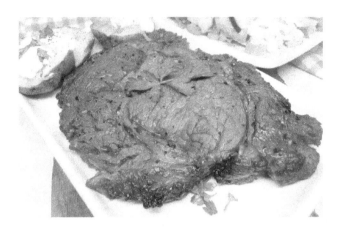

Method

1. Mix olive oil, soy sauce, seasoning and steaks in a clean bowl and set aside meat for marination.

2. Take out steaks and waste the remaining mixture. Remove excess oil from steak by patting.

3. Add 1 tablespoon water in an air fryer pot for the prevention from smoking during cooking of steaks.

3. Set the temperature of an air fryer to 200C. Place steaks in an air fryer pot. Air fry for 7-8 minutes and turn its side after every 8 minutes. Cook for more 7 minutes until it is rarely medium. Cook for final 3 minutes for a medium steak and dish out in a clean plate and serve immediately.

29. Air Fried Potato Chips

Ingredients

- Large potatoes - 2
- Olive oil - to spray
- Fresh parsley - optional
- Sea salt - 1/2 teaspoon

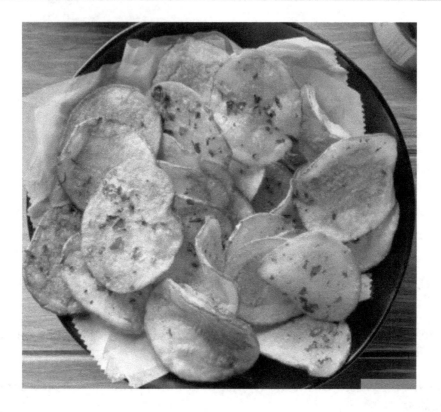

Method

1. Set the temperature of an air fryer to 180C.

2. Peel off the potatoes and cut them into thin slices. Shift the slices in a bowl containing ice chilled water and soak for 10 minutes. Drain potatoes, again add chilled water and soak for more 15 minutes.

3. Remove water from potatoes and allow to dry by using paper towel. Spray potatoes with cooking oil and add salt according to taste.

4. Place a single layer of potatoes slices in an oiled air fryer pot and cook for 15-18 minutes until color turns to golden brown and crispy. Stir constantly and turn its sides after every 5 minutes.

5. Dish out these crispy chips and serve with parsley.

30. Air Fried Tofu

Ingredients

- Packed tofu - 14 ounces
- Olive oil - 1/4 cup
- Reduced sodium soy sauce - 3 tablespoons

- Crushed red pepper flakes - 1/4 teaspoon
- Green onions - 2
- Cumin powder - 1/4 teaspoon
- Garlic - 2 cloves

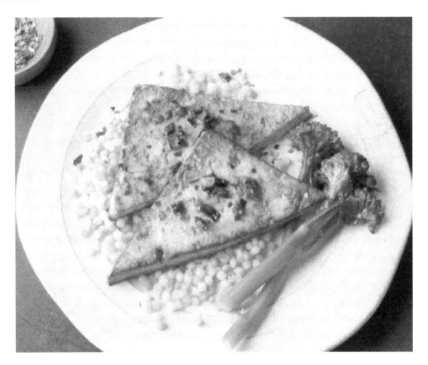

Method

1. Set the temperature of an air fryer to 200C.

2. Mix olive oil, soy sauce, onions, garlic, cumin powder and red pepper flakes in a deep bowl to make marinade mixture.

3. Cut 3/8 inches' thick slices of tofu lengthwise and then diagonally. Coat tofu with marinade mixture. Place them in refrigerate for 4-5 minutes and turn them after every 2 minutes.

4. Place tofu in buttered air fryer pot. Put remaining marinade over each tofu. Cook for 5-8 minutes until color turns to golden brown. Dish out cooked tofu and serve immediately.

31. Air Fried Acorn Squash Slices

Ingredients

- Medium sized acorn squash - 2
- Soft butter - 1/2 cup

- Brown sugar - 2/3 cup

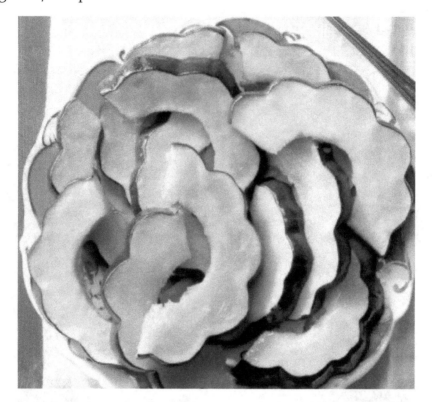

Method

1. Set the temperature of an air fryer to 160C.

2. Cut squash into two halves from length side and remove seeds. Again cut these halves into half inch slices.

3. Place a single layer of squash on buttered air fryer pot. Cook each side of squash for 5 minutes.

4. Mix butter into brown sugar and spread this mixture on the top of every squash. Cook for more 3 minutes. Dish out and serve immediately.

32. Air Fried Red Potatoes

Ingredients

- Baby potatoes - 2 pounds
- Olive oil - 2 tablespoons
- Fresh rosemary - 1 tablespoon
- Garlic - 2 cloves
- Salt - 1/2 teaspoon

- Black pepper - 1/4 teaspoon

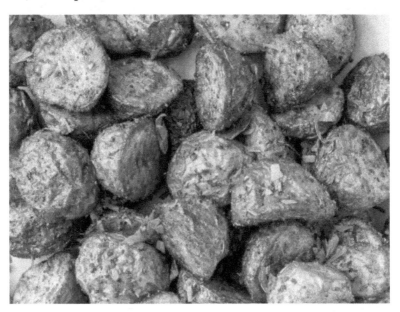

Method

1. Set the temperature of an air fryer to 198C.

2. Cut potatoes into wedges. Coat them properly with minced garlic, rosemary, black pepper and salt.

3. Place coated potatoes on buttered air fryer pot. Cook potatoes for 5 minutes until golden brown and soft. Stir them at once. Dish out in a clean plate and serve immediately.

33. Air Fried Butter Cake

Ingredients

- Melted butter - 7 tablespoons
- White sugar - 1/4 cup & 2 tablespoons
- Plain flour - 1 & 2/3 cup
- Egg - 1
- Salt - 1 pinch
- Milk - 6 tablespoons
- Cooking oil - to spray

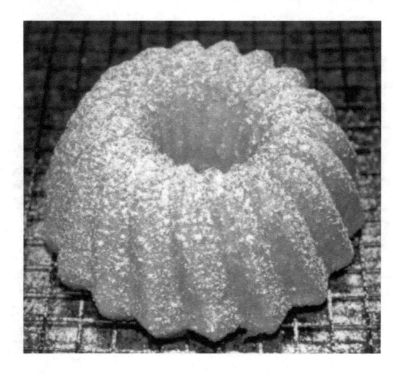

Method

1. Set the temperature of an air fryer to 180C and spray with cooking oil.

2. Beat white sugar, and butter together in a clean bowl until creamy and light. Then add egg and beautiful fluffy and smooth. Add salt and flour and stir. Then add milk and mix until batter is smooth. Shift batter to an preheated air fryer pot and level its surface by using spatula.

3. Place in an air fryer and set time of 15 minutes. Bake and check cake after 15 minutes by inserting toothpick in the cake. If toothpick comes out clean it means cake has fully baked.

4. Take out cake from air fryer and allow it to cool for 5-10 minutes. Serve immediately and enjoy.

34. Air Fried Jelly and Peanut Butter S'mores

Ingredients

- Chocolate topping peanut butter cup - 1
- Raspberry jam (seedless) - 1 teaspoon
- Marshmallow - 1 large
- Chocolate cracker squares – 2

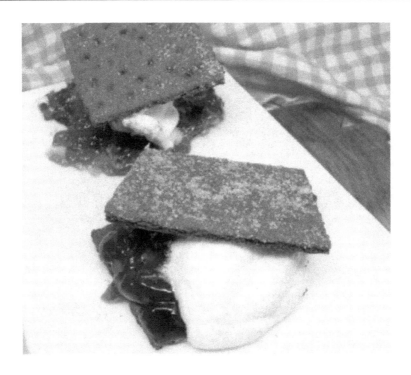

Method

1. Set the temperature of an air fryer to 200C.

2. Put peanut butter cup on one cracker square and topped with marshmallow and jelly. Carefully transfer it in the preheated air fryer.

3. Cook for 1 minute until marshmallow becomes soft and light brown. Remaining cracker squares is used for topping.

4. Shift this delicious in a clean plate and serve immediately.

35. Air Fried Sun-Dried Tomatoes

Ingredients

- Red grape tomatoes - 5 ounces
- Olive oil - 1/4 teaspoon
- Salt - to taste

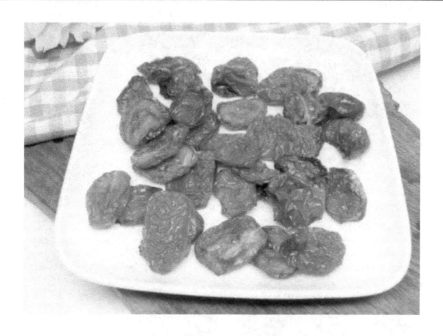

Method

1. Set the temperature of an air fryer to 115C.

2. Combine tomatoes halves, salt and olive oil evenly in a clean bowl. Shift tomatoes in an air fryer pot by placing skin side down.

3. Cook in air fryer for 45 minutes. Smash tomatoes by using spatula and cook for more 30 minutes. Repeat this step with the rest of tomatoes.

4. Shift this delicious dish in a clean plate and allow it to stand for 45 minutes to set. Serve this dish and enjoy.

36. Air Fried Sweet Potatoes Tots

Ingredients:

- Peeled Sweet Potatoes - 2 small (14oz.total)
- Garlic Powder - 1/8 tsp
- Potato Starch - 1 tbsp
- Kosher Salt, Divided - 11/4 tsp
- Unsalted Ketchup - 3/4 Cup
- Cooking Oil for spray

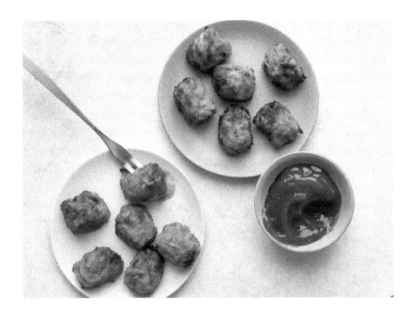

Method:

1. Take water in a medium pan and give a single boil over high flame. Then, add the sweet potatoes in the boiled water & cook for 15 minutes till potatoes becomes soft. Move the potatoes to a cooling plate for 15 minutes.

2. Rub potatoes using the wide hole's grater over a dish. Apply the potato starch, salt and garlic powder and toss gently. Make almost 24 shaped cylinders (1-inch) from the mixture.

3. Coat the air fryer pot gently with cooking oil. Put single layer of 1/2 of the tots in the pot and spray with cooking oil. Cook at 400 °F for about 12 to 14 minutes till lightly browned and flip tots midway. Remove from the pot and sprinkle with salt. Repeat with rest of the tots and salt left over. Serve with ketchup immediately.

37. Air Fried Banana Bread

Ingredients:

- White Whole Wheat Flour - 3/4 cup (3 oz.)
- Mashed Ripe Bananas - 2 medium or (about 3/4th cup)
- Cinnamon powder– 4 pinches
- Kosher Salt - 1/2 tsp
- Baking Soda - 1/4 tsp
- Large Eggs, Lightly Beaten - 2
- Regular Sugar - 1/2 cup
- Vanilla Essence - 1 tsp
- Vegetable Oil - 2 tbsp
- Roughly Chopped and toasted Walnuts - 2 table-spoons (3/4 oz.)

- Plain Non-Fat Yogurt - 1/3 cup
- Cooking Oil for Spray - as required

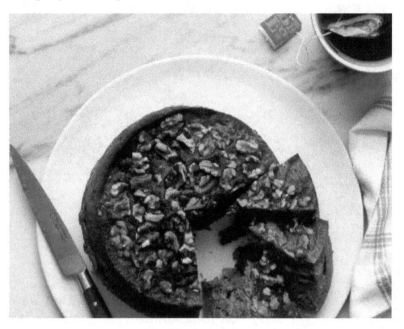

Method:

1. Cover the base of a 6-inches round cake baking pan with baking paper and lightly brush with melted butter. Beat the flour, baking soda, salt, and cinnamon together in a clean bowl and let it reserve.

2. Whisk the mashed bananas, eggs, sugar, cream, oil and vanilla together in a separate bowl. Stir the wet ingredients gently into the flour mixture until everything is blended. Pour the mixture in the prepared pan and sprinkle with the walnuts.

3. Set the temperature of an air fryer to 310 °F and put the pan in the air fryer. Cook until browned, about 30 to 35 minutes. Rotate the pan periodically until a wooden stick put in it and appears clean. Before flipping out & slicing, move the bread to a cooling rack for 15 minutes.

38. Air Fried Avocado Fries

Ingredients:

- Avocados --. 2 - Cut each into the 8 pieces
- All-purpose flour - 1/2 cup (about 21/8 oz.)
- Panko (Japanese Style Breadcrumbs) - 1/2 cup
- Large Eggs - 2
- Kosher Salt - 1/4 tsp
- Apple Cider - 1 tbsp

- Sriracha Chilli Sause - 1 tbsp
- Black pepper - 11/2 tsp
- Water - 1 tbsp
- Unsalted Ketchup - 1/2 cup
- Cooking spray

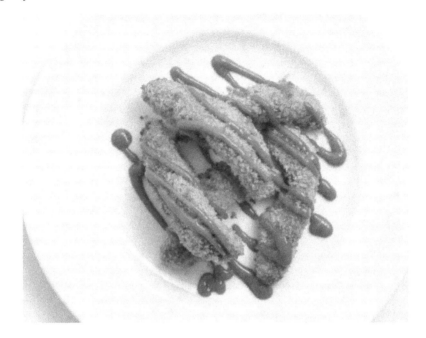

Method:

1. Mix flour and pepper collectively in a clean bowl. Whip eggs & water gently in another bowl. Take panko in a third bowl. Coat avocado slices in flour and remove extra flour by shaking. Then, dip the slices in the egg and remove any excess. Coat in panko by pushing to stick together. Spray well the avocado slices with cooking oil.

2. In the air fryer's basket, put avocado slices & fry at 400 ° F until it turns into golden for 7-8 minutes. Turn avocado wedges periodically while frying. Take out from an air fryer and use salt for sprinkling.

3. Mix the Sriracha, ketchup, vinegar, and mayonnaise together in a small bowl. Put two tablespoons of sauce on each plate with 4 avocado fries before serving.

39. "Strawberry Pop Tarts" in an Air Fryer

Ingredients:

- Quartered Strawberries - (about 13/4 cups equal to 8 ounces)
- White/Regular Sugar - 1/4 cup
- Refrigerated Piecrusts - 1/2(14.1-oz)

- Powdered Sugar - 1/2 cup (about 2-oz)
- Fresh Lemon Juice - 11/2 tsp
- Rainbow Candy Sprinkles - 1 tbsp(about 1/2 ounce)
- Cooking Spray

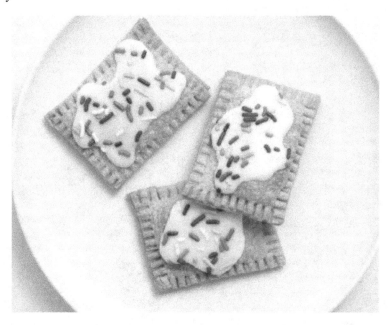

Method:

1. Mix strawberries & white sugar and stay for 15 minutes with periodically stirring. Air fryer them for 10 minutes until glossy and reduced with constant stirring. Let it cool for 30 minutes.

2. Use the smooth floured surface to roll the pie crust and make 12-inches round shape. Cut the dough into 12 rectangles of (2 1/2- x 3-inch), re-rolling strips if necessary. Leaving a 1/2-inch boundary, add the spoon around 2 tea-spoons of strawberry mixture into the middle of 6 of dough rectangles. Brush the edges of the rectangles of the filled dough with water. Then, press the edges of rest dough rectangles with a fork to seal. Spray the tarts very well with cooking oil.

3. In an air fryer pot, put 3 tarts in a single layer and cook them at 350 ° F for 10 minutes till golden brown. With the rest of the tarts, repeat the process. Set aside for cooling for 30 minutes.

4. In a small cup, whip the powdered sugar & lemon juice together until it gets smooth. Glaze the spoon over the cooled tarts and sprinkle equally with candy.

40. Lighten up Empanadas in an Air Fryer

Ingredients:

- Lean Green Beef - 3 ounces
- Cremini Mushrooms - Chopped finely - 3 ounces
- White onion - Chopped finely - 1/4th cup
- Garlic – Chopped finely - 2 tsp.
- Pitted Green Olives - 6
- Olive Oil - 1 table-spoon
- Cumin - 1/4th tsp
- Cinnamon - 1/8th tsp
- Chopped tomatoes - 1/2 cup
- Paprika - 1/4 tea-spoon
- Large egg lightly Beaten - 1
- Square gyoza wrappers - 8

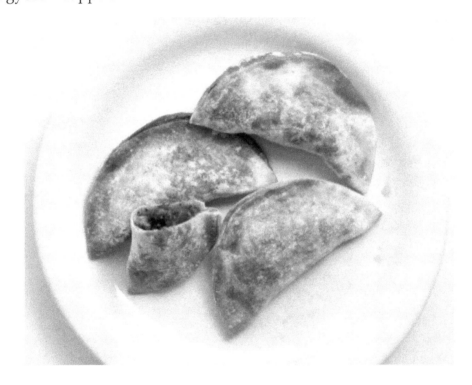

Method:

1. In a medium cooking pot, let heat oil on the medium/high temperature. Then, add beef & onion; for 3 minutes, cook them, mixing the crumble, until getting brown. Put the mushrooms; let them cook for 6 mins, till the mushrooms start to brown, stirring frequently. Add the paprika, olives, garlic, cinnamon, and cumin; cook for three minutes until the mushrooms are very tender and most of the liquid has been released. Mix in the tomatoes and cook, turning periodically, for 1 minute. Put the filling in a bowl and let it cool for 5 minutes.

2. Arrange 4 wrappers of gyoza on a worktop. In each wrapper, put around 1 1/2 tablespoons of filling in the middle. Clean the edges of the egg wrappers; fold over the

wrappers and pinch the edges to seal. Repeat with the remaining wrappers and filling process.

3. Place the 4 empanadas in one single layer in an air-fryer basket and cook for 7 minutes at 400 °F until browned well. Repeat with the empanadas that remain.

41. Air Fried Calzones

Ingredients:

- Spinach Leaves --> 3 ounces (about 3 cups)
- Shredded Chicken breast --> 2 ounces (about 1/3 cup)
- Fresh Whole Wheat Pizza Dough --> 6 ounces
- Shredded Mozzarella Cheese --> 1 1/2 ounces (about 6 tbsp)
- Low Sodium Marinara Sauce --> 1/3 cup

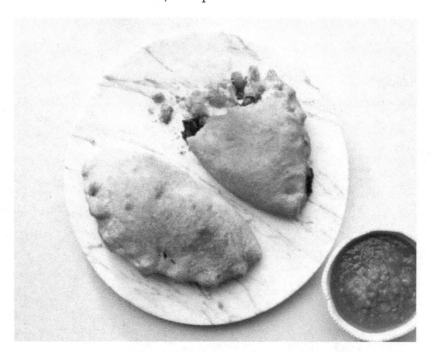

Method:

1. First of all, in a medium pan, let heat oil on medium/high temperature. Include onion & cook, continue mixing then well efficiently, for two min, till get soft. After that, add the spinach; then cover & cook it until softened. After that, take out the pan from the heat; mix the chicken & marinara sauce.

2. Divide the dough in to the four identical sections. Then, roll each section into a 6-inches circle on a gently floured surface. Place over half of each dough circular shape with one-fourth of the spinach mixture. Top with one-fourth of the cheese each. Fold

the dough to make half-moons and over filling, tightening the edges to lock. Coat the calzones well with spray for cooking

3. In the basket of an air fryer, put the calzones and cook them at 325 ° F until the dough becomes nicely golden brown, in 12 mins, changing the sides of the calzones after 8 mins.

42. Air Fried Mexican Style Corns

Ingredients:

- Unsalted Butter - 11/2 tbsp.
- Chopped Garlic -2 tsp
- Shucked Fresh Corns - 11/2 lb
- Fresh Chopped Cilantro - 2 tbsp.
- Lime zest - 1 tbsp.
- Lime Juice - 1 tsp
- Kosher Salt - 1/2 tsp
- Black Pepper - 1/2 tsp

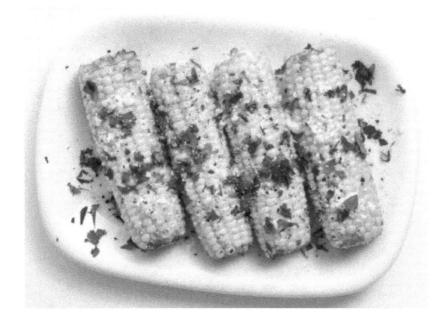

Method:

1. Coat the corn delicately with the cooking spray, and put the corn in the air fryer's basket in one single layer. Let it Cooking for 14 mins at 400 °F till tender then charred gently, changing the corn half the way via cooking.

2. In the meantime, whisk together all the garlic, lime juice, butter, & lime zest in the microwaveable pot. Let an air fryer on Fast, about 30 seconds, until the butter melts and

the garlic is aromatic. Put the corn on the plate and drop the butter mixture on it. Using the salt, cilantro, and pepper to sprinkle. Instantly serve this delicious recipe.

43. Air Fryer Crunchy & Crispy Chocolate Bites

Ingredients:

- Frozen Shortcrust Pastry - Partially thawed -- 4
- Cinnamon for dusting -- as required
- Icing Sugar for dusting -- as required
- Mars Celebration Chocolates -- 24
- Whipped Cream - as required

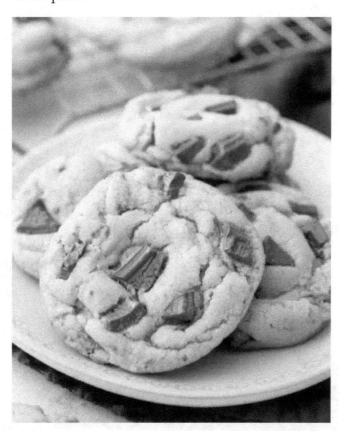

Method:

1. First of all, cut each pastry sheet into 6 equal rectangles. Brush the egg finely. In the centre of each piece of the pastry, place one chocolate. Fold the pastry over to seal the chocolate. Trim the extra pastry, then press and lock the corners. Put it on a tray lined with baking sheet. Brush the tops with an egg. Use the mixture of cinnamon and sugar to sprinkle liberally.

2. In the air-fryer basket, put a layer of the baking paper, ensuring that the paper is 1 cm smaller than that of the basket to permit air to circulate well. Place the 6 pockets in basket, taking care that these pockets must not to overlap. Then, cook them for 8-9 mins at 190 ° C till they become golden and the pastry are prepared thoroughly. As the pockets cooked, transfer them into a dish. Repeat the process with the pockets that remain.

3. After taking out from the air fryer, dust the Icing sugar and at last with whipped cream. Serve them warm.

44. Doritos-Crumbled Chicken tenders in an Air fryer

Ingredients:

- Buttermilk -- 1 cup (about 250ml)
- Doritos Nacho Cheese Corn Chips -- 170g Packet
- Halved Crossways Chicken Tenderloins -- 500g
- Egg -- 1
- Plain Flour -- 50g
- Mild Salsa -- for serving

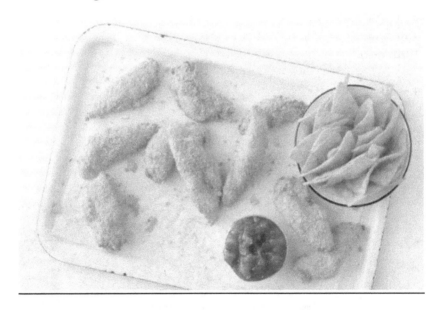

Method:

1.Take a ceramic bowl or glass and put the chicken in it. Then, c over the buttermilk with it. Wrap it and put it for 4 hours or may be overnight in the refrigerator to marinate.

2. Let Preheat an air fryer at 180C. Then, cover a Baking tray with grease-proof paper.

3. In a Chopper, add the corn chips then pulse them until the corn chips become coarsely chopped. Then, transfer the chopped chips to a dish. In a deep cup, put the egg and beat it. On another plate, put the flour.

4. Remove the unnecessary water from the chicken, and also discard the buttermilk. Then, dip the chicken in the flour mixture and wipe off the extra flour. After that, dip in the beaten egg and then into the chips of corn, press it firmly to coat well. Transfer it to the tray that made ready to next step.

5. In the air fryer, put half of the chicken and then, fry for 8 to 10 mins until they are golden as well as cooked completely. Repeat the process with the chicken that remain.

Transfer the chicken in the serving dish. Enjoy this delicious recipe with salsa.

45. Air Fryer Ham & Cheese Croquettes

Ingredients:

- Chopped White Potatoes -- 1 kg
- Chopped Ham -- 100g
- Chopped Green Shallots -- 2
- Grated Cheddar Cheese -- 80g (about 1 cup)
- All-purpose flour -- 50g
- eggs -- 2
- Breadcrumbs -- 100g
- Lemon Slices -- for serving
- Tonkatsu Sause -- for serving

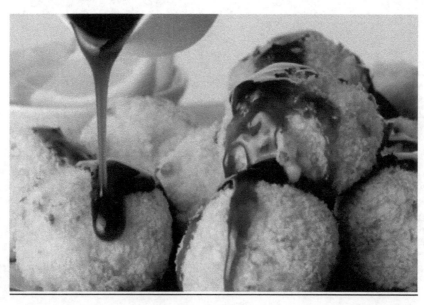

Method:

1. In a large-sized saucepan, put the potatoes. Cover with chill water. Carry it over high temperature to a boil. Boil till tender for 10 to 12 minutes. Drain thoroughly. Return over low heat to pan. Mix until it is smooth and has allowed to evaporate the certain water. Withdraw from the sun. Switch to a tub. Fully set aside to chill.

2. Then, add the shallot, Ham and cheese in the mashed potatoes also season with kosher salt. Mix it well. Take the 2 tablespoons of the mixture and make its balls. And repeat process for the rest of mixture.

3. Take the plain flour in a plate. Take another small bowl and beat the eggs. Take the third bowl and add the breadcrumbs in it. Toss the balls in the flour. Shake off the extra flour then in eggs and coat the breadcrumbs well. Make the balls ready for frying. Take all the coated balls in the fridge for about 15 minutes.

4. Preheat an air fryer at 200 ° C. Then, cook the croquettes for 8 to10 mints until they become nicely golden, in two rounds. Sprinkle the tonkatsu sauce and serve the croquettes with lemon slices.

46. Air Fryer Lemonade Scones

Ingredients:

- Self-raising flour -- 525g (about 3 1/2 cups)
- Thickened Cream -- 300ml
- Lemonade -- 185ml (about 3/4 cup)
- Caster Sugar -- 70g (1/3 cup)
- Vanilla Essence -- 1 tsp
- Milk -- for brushing
- Raspberry Jam -- for serving
- Whipped Cream -- for serving

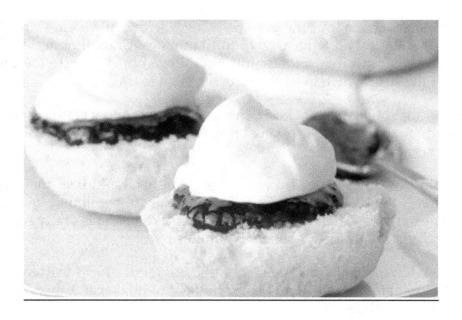

Method:

1. In a large-sized bowl, add the flour and sugar together. Mix it well. Add lemonade, vanilla and cream. In a big bowl, add the flour and sugar. Just make a well. Remove milk, vanilla and lemonade. Mix finely, by using a plain knife, till the dough comes at once.

2. Take out the dough on the flat surface and sprinkle the dry flour on the dough. Knead it gently for about 30 secs until the dough get smooth. On a floured surface, roll out the dough. Politely knead for thirty seconds, until it is just smooth. Form the dough into a round shape about 2.5 cm thick. Toss around 5.5 cm blade into the flour. Cut the scones out. Push the bits of remaining dough at once gently and repeat the process to make Sixteen scones.

3. In the air fryer bucket, put a layer of baking paper, ensuring that the paper is 1 cm shorter than the bucket to allow air to flow uniformly. Put 5 to 6 scones on paper in the bucket, even hitting them. Finely brush the surfaces with milk. Let cook them for about 15 mins at 160 ° C or when they tapped on the top, until become golden and empty-sounding. Move it safely to a wire or cooling rack. Repeat the same process with the rest of scones and milk two more times.

4. Serve the lemonade scones warm with raspberry jam & whipped cream.

47. Air Fryer Baked Potatoes

Ingredients:

- Baby Potatoes -- Halved shape -- 650g
- Fresh rosemary sprigs-- 2 large
- Sour Cream -- for serving

- Sweet Chilli Sauce -- for serving
- Salt -- for seasoning

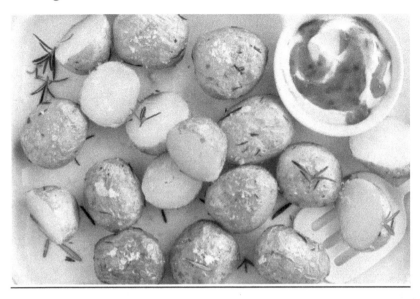

Method:

1. Firstly, at 180C, pre-heat the air fryer. In an air fryer, put the rosemary sprigs & baby potatoes. Use oil for spray and salt for seasoning. Then, cook them for fifteen min until become crispy and cooked completely, also turning partially.

2. Serve the baked potatoes sweet chilli Sause & sour cream to enhance its flavour.

48. Air Fryer Mozzarella Chips

Ingredients:

- All-purpose flour -- 1 tbsp
- Breadcrumbs -- 2/3 cup
- Garlic Powder -- 3 tbsp
- Lemon Juice -- 1/3 cup
- Avocado -- 1
- Basil Pesto -- 2 tbsp
- Plain Yogurt -- 1/4 cup
- Chopped Green Onion --1
- Cornflakes crumbs -- 1/4 cup
- Mozzarella block -- 550g
- Eggs – 2
- Olive Oil for spray

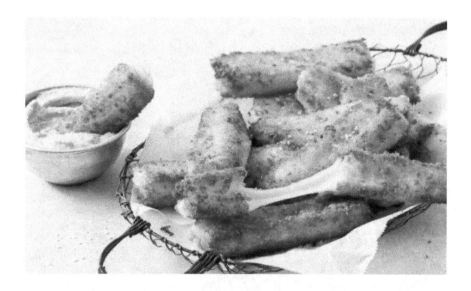

Method:

1. Start making Creamy and fluffy Avocado Dipped Sauce: In a small-sized food processor, put the yogurt, avocado, lemon juice, onion, and pesto. Also add the pepper & salt, blend properly. Process it well until it get mixed and smooth. Switch the batter to a bowl. Cover it. Place in the fridge, until It required.

2. Take a large-sized tray and place a baking sheet. In a large bowl, add the garlic powder & plain flour together. Also add the salt and season well. Take another medium bowl, whisk the eggs. Mix the breadcrumbs well in bowl.

3. Make the 2 cm thick wedges of mozzarella, then put them into the sticks. For coating, roll the cheese in the flour. Shake off the extra flour. Then, coat the sticks in the egg fusion, then in the breadcrumbs, operating in rounds. Place the prepared plate on it. Freeze till solid, or even for around 1 hour.

4. Spray the oil on the mozzarella lightly. Wrap the air fryer bucket with baking sheet, leaving an edge of 1 cm to enable air to flow. Then, cook at 180C, for 4 to 4 1/2 mins until the sticks become crispy & golden. Serve warm with sauce to dip.

49. Air Fryer Fetta Nuggets

Ingredients:

- All-purpose flour -- 1 tbsp.
- Chilli flakes -- 1 tsp
- Onion powder -- 1 tsp
- Sesame Seeds -- 1/4 cup
- Fetta Cheese Cubes -- Cut in 2 cm 180g
- Fresh Chives -- for serving

- Breadcrumbs -- 1/4 cup

BARBECUE SAUSE:

- apple cider -- 11/2 tsp
- Chilli Flakes -- 1/2 tsp
- Barbecue Sause -- 1//4 cup

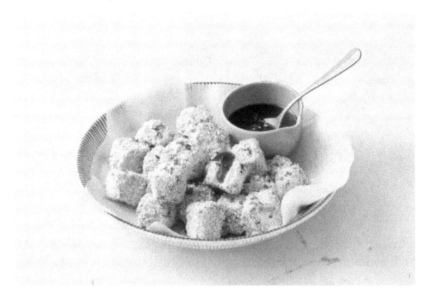

Method:

1. Mix the onion powder, flour and chilli flakes in a medium-sized bowl. Use pepper for seasoning. Take another bowl, and beat an egg. Take one more bowl and mix sesame seeds and breadcrumbs. Then, toss the fetta in the chilli flakes, onion powder & flour mixture. Dip the fetta in egg, and toss again in breadcrumbs fusion. Put them on a plate.

2. Pre- heat the air fryer at 180 °C. Put the cubes of fetta in a baking tray, in the basket of the air fryer. cook till fetta cubes become golden, or may be for 6 mins.

3. In the meantime, mix all the wet ingredients and create the Barbecue sauce.

4. Sprinkle the chives on the fetta and serve with Barbecue Sause.

50. Air Fryer Japanese Chicken Tender

Ingredients:

- McCormick Katsu Crumb for seasoning -- 25g
- Pickled Ginger -- 1 tbsp.
- Japanese-Style Mayonnaise -- 1/3 cup
- Chicken Tenderloins -- 500g

- Oil for spray

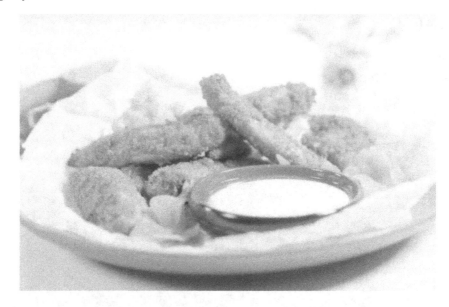

Method:

1. Put the chicken on tray in the form of single layer. Sprinkle the half seasoning on chicken. Then, turn chicken and sprinkle the seasoning again evenly. Use oil for spray on it.

2. Pre-heat at 180°C, an air fryer. Let the chicken cooking for about 12 - 14 mins until it becomes golden & cooked completely.

3. In the meantime, take a small-sized bowl, mix the mayonnaise and the remaining pickling sauce.

4. Serve the chicken with white sauce and put the ginger on the side, in a platter.

51. Whole-Wheat Pizzas in an Air Fryer

Ingredients:

- Low-sodium Marinara Sauce -- 1/4 cup
- Spinach leaves -- 1 cup
- Pita Breads -- 2
- Shredded Mozzarella Cheese -- 1/4 cup
- Parmigiano- Reggiano Cheese -- 1/4 ounces (about 1 tbsp.)
- Tomato slices -- 8
- Sliced Garlic Clove -- 1

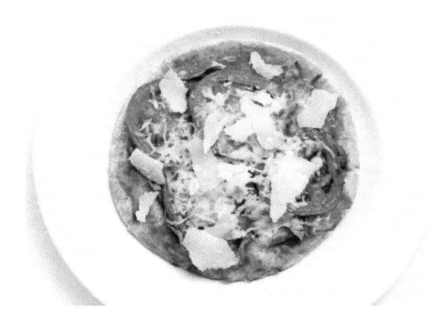

Method:

1. Spread the marinara sauce on 1 side of each pita bread uniformly. Cover the cheese spinach leaves, tomato slices and garlic, with half of each of these.

2. Put one pita bread in an air fryer pot, then cook it at 350°F till the cheese becomes melted and pita becomes crispy, 4 - 5 mins. Repeat the process with the pita leftover.

52. Air Fryer Crispy Veggie Quesadillas

Ingredients:

- 6 inches Whole Grain Flour Tortillas -- 4
- Full fat Cheddar Cheese -- 4 ounces (about 1 cup)
- Sliced Zucchini -- 1 cup
- Lime Zest -- 1 tbsp.
- Lime Juice -- 1 tsp.
- Fresh Cilantro -- 2 tbsp.
- Chopped Red Bell Pepper -- (about 1 cup)
- Cumin -- 1/4 tsp.
- Low-fat Yoghurt -- 2 ounces
- Refrigerated Pico de Gallo -- 1/2 cup
- Oil for spray

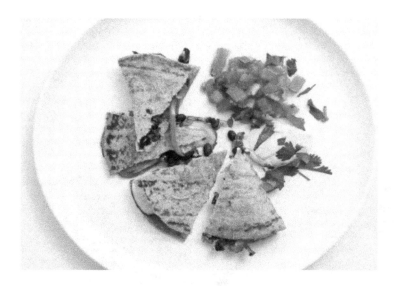

Method:

1. Put tortillas on the surface of the work. Sprinkle onto half of each tortilla with 2 tbsp. of grated cheese. Cover each tortilla with 1/4 cup of chopped red bell pepper, zucchini chunks & the black beans on the top of the cheese. Sprinkle finely with 1/2 cup of cheese left. Fold over the tortillas to create quesadillas form like half-moons. Coat the quesadillas slightly with a cooking spray, & lock them with match picks or toothpicks.

2. Lightly brush a bucket of air fryer with cooking oil spray. Place 2 quesadillas carefully in the basket. Cook at 400°F till the tortillas become golden brown & gently crispy. Melt the cheese & gradually tender the vegetables for ten mins, tossing the quesadillas partially throughout the cooking period. Repeat the process with leftover quesadillas.

3. Mix together lime zest, yogurt, cumin, & lime juice, in a small-sized bowl since the quesadillas getting prepare. Break each quesadilla in-to the pieces to serve and then sprinkle the coriander. With one tbsp. of cumin cream and two tablespoons of pico de gallo, and serve each.

53. Air Fried Curry Chickpeas

Ingredients:

- Drained & Rinsed Un-Salted Chickpeas -- 11/2 cups (15-oz.)
- Olive Oil -- 2 tbsp.
- Curry Powder -- 2 tsp.
- Coriander -- 1/4 tsp.
- Cumin -- 1/4 tsp.
- Cinnamon -- 1/4 tsp.
- Turmeric -- 1/2 tsp.
- Aleppo Pepper -- 1/2 tsp.

- Red Wine Vinegar -- 2 tbsp.
- Kosher Salt -- 1/4 tsp.
- Sliced Fresh Cilantro -- as required

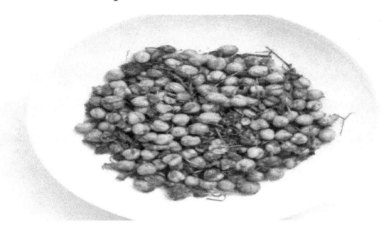

Method:

1. Break the chickpeas lightly in a medium-sized bowl with your hands (don't crush them); and then remove the skins of chickpea.

2. Add oil & vinegar to the chickpeas, and stir to coat. Then, add curry powder, turmeric, coriander, cumin, & cinnamon; mix gently to combine them.

3. In the air fryer bucket, put the chickpeas in one single layer & cook at 400°F temperature until becoming crispy, for about 15 min, stirring the chickpeas periodically throughout the cooking process.

4. Place the chickpeas in a dish. Sprinkle the salt, cilantro and Aleppo pepper on chickpeas; and cover it.

54. Air Fried Beet Chips

Ingredients:

- Canola Oil -- 1 tsp.
- Medium-sized Red Beets -- 3
- Black Pepper -- 1/4 tsp.
- Kosher Salt -- 3/4 tsp.

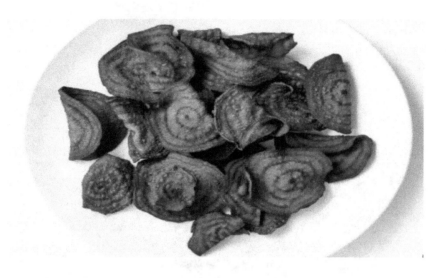

Method:

1. Cut and Peel the red beets. Make sure each beet cutted into 1/8-inch-thick slices. Take a large-sized bowl and toss the beets slices, pepper, salt and oil well.

2. Put half beets in air fryer bucket and then cook at the 320°F temperature about 25 - 30 mins or until they become crispy and dry. Flip the bucket about every 5 mins. Repeat the process for the beets that remain.

55. Double-Glazed Air Fried Cinnamon Biscuits

Ingredients:

- Cinnamon -- 1/4 tsp.
- Plain Flour -- 2/3 cup (about 27/8 oz.)
- Whole-Wheat Flour -- 2/3 cup (about22/3 oz.)
- Baking Powder -- 1 tsp.
- White Sugar -- 2 tbsp.
- Kosher Salt -- 1/4 tsp.
- Chill Salted Butter -- 4 tbsp.
- Powdered Sugar -- 2 cups (about 8-oz.)
- Water -- 3 tbsp.
- Whole Milk -- 1/3 cup
- Oil for spray -- as required

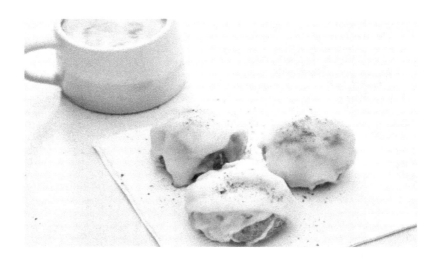

Method:

1. In a medium-sized bowl, stir together salt, plain flour, baking powder, white sugar cinnamon and butter. Use two knives or pastry cutter to cut mixture till butter becomes well mixed with the flour and the mixture seems to as coarse cornmeal. Add the milk, then mix well until the dough becomes a ball. Place the dough on a floury surface and knead for around 30 seconds until the dough becomes smooth. Break the dough into 16 identical parts. Roll each part carefully into a plain ball.

2. Coat the air fryer pot well with oil spray. Put 8 balls in the pot, by leaving the space between each one; spray with cooking oil. Cook them until get browned & puffed, for 10 - 12 mins at 350°F temperature. Take out the doughnut balls from the pot carefully and put them on a cooling rack having foil for five mins. Repeat the process with the doughnut balls that remain.

3. In a medium pot, mix water and powdered sugar together until smooth. Then, spoon half of the glaze carefully over the doughnut balls. Cool for five mins and let it glaze once and enabling to drip off extra glaze.

56. Lemon Drizzle Cake in an Air Fryer

Ingredients:

- Grated Lemon rind -- 2 tsp.
- Cardamom -- 1 tsp.
- Softened Butter -- 150g
- Eggs -- 3
- Honey-flavoured Yoghurt -- 3/4 cup
- Self-raising flour -- 11/2 cups
- Caster Sugar -- 2/3 cup (150g)
- Lemon Zest -- for serving

LEMON ICING:

- Icing Sugar -- 1 cup
- Lemon Juice -- 11/2 tbsps.
- Softened Butter -- 10g

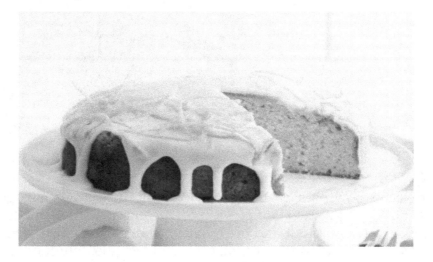

Method:

1. First, grease a 20 cm cake baking pan of round shape having butter paper. Take an electric beater and beat cardamom, sugar, lemon rind, and butter until the mixture becomes smooth & pale. Then, add the eggs one by one and beat well. Put the eggs in the flour and yoghurt. Fold by spatula and make the surface very smooth.

2. Pre-heat the air fryer at 180 C temperature. Put the pan in air fryer's pot. Bake it for about 35 mins. Check it by putting skewer in it that comes out clean without any sticky batter. Reserve it in the pan for 5 minutes to become cool before shifting it to a cooling rack.

3. Make the lemon glaze, add butter and icing sugar in a bowl. By adding lemon juice as required and form a smooth paste.

4. Put the cake on a plate to serve. Sprinkle the lemon zest and lemon icing to serve.

57. Air Fryer dukkah-Crumbed chicken

Ingredients:

- Chicken Thigh Fillets -- 8
- Herb or dukkah -- 45g packet
- Plain Flour -- 1/3 cup (about 50g)
- Kaleslaw kit -- 350g Packet
- Breadcrumbs -- 1 cup (about 80g)

- Eggs -- 2

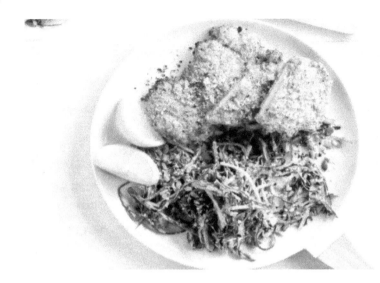

Method:

1. Put half of the chicken within 2 sheets of cling paper. Gently beat until it remains 2 cm thick by using a meat hammer or rolling pin. Repeat the process with the chicken that remains.

2. In a deep bowl, mix breadcrumbs and dukkah together. Beat an egg in medium bowl., Put the flour and all the seasoning on a tray. Coat chicken pieces one by one in the flour and shake off the extra. Dip chicken pieces into the egg, then in breadcrumbs for coating. Move them to a dish. Cover them with the plastic wrapper & leave it to marinate for 30 mins in the fridge.

3. Pre-heat air fryer at 200°C temperature. Use olive oil to spray the chicken pieces. Put half of the chicken in one single layer in the air fryer pot. Cook them for about 16 mins and turning partially until they become golden & get cooked completely. Move to a plate & wrap them with foil to stay warm. Repeat the process with the chicken pieces that remains.

4. After that, place the kaleslaw kit in a serving bowl by following instructions mentioned in the packets.

5. Divide the prepared chicken & the kaleslaw between serving platters, and season it.

58. Air Fryer Vietnamese-style spring roll salad

Ingredients:

- Rice Noodles -- 340g
- Crushed Garlic -- 1 clove

- Grated Ginger -- 2 tsp.
- Pork Mince -- 250g
- Lemongrass paste -- 1 tsp
- Cutted into matchsticks the Peeled Carrots -- 2
- Sliced Spring onion -- 3
- Fish sauce -- 2 tsp.
- Spring roll pastries -- 10 sheets
- Coriander -- 1/2 cup
- Sliced Red Chilli - 1 long
- Vietnamese-style Salad -- for dressing
- Mint Leaves -- 1/2
- Bean Sprouts -- 1 cup

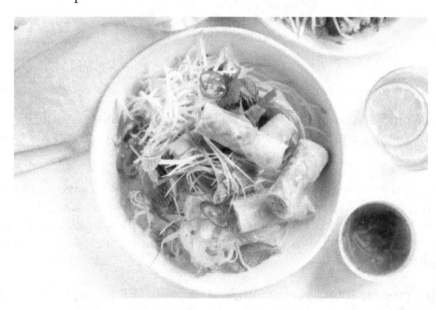

Method:

1. Take a large-sized saucepan and cook the noodles for about 4 mins until get soft. Take the cold water and discharge thoroughly. Cutting 1 cup of the boiled noodles into the short lengths, with the leftover noodles reserved.

2. Take a large-sized bowl, add the mince, lemongrass, ginger, garlic, half carrot, spring onion, and fish sauce together and mix them well.

3. On a clean surface, put one pastry paper. Add two tablespoons across 1 side of the mince fusion diagonally. With just a little spray, brush its opposite side. Fold and roll on the sides to completely cover the mince filling. Repeat the process with the sheets of pastry and fill the thin layer of mince mixture, that remain.

4. Pre-heat at 200°C, an air fryer. Use olive oil, spray on the spring rolls. Put in the bucket of air fryer and cook the spring rolls for fifteen mins until cooked completely. Change the sides half-way during cooking.

5. After that, equally split reserved noodles in the serving bowls. Place coriander, bean sprouts, mint and the remaining spring onion and carrots at the top of the serving bowl.

6. Then, break the spring rolls in the half and place them over the mixture of noodles. Sprinkle the chili and serve with Vietnamese-style salad dressing according to your taste.

59. Air Fryer Pizza Pockets

Ingredients:

- Olive oil - 2 tsp.
- Sliced Mushrooms - 6 (about 100g)
- Chopped Leg Ham - 50g
- Crumbled Fetta - 80g
- White Wraps - 4
- Basil Leaves - 1/4 cup
- Baby Spinach - 120g
- Tomato Paste - 1/3 cup
- Chopped Red Capsicum - 1/2
- Dried Oregano - 1/2 tsp
- Olive oil - for spray
- Green Salad - for serving

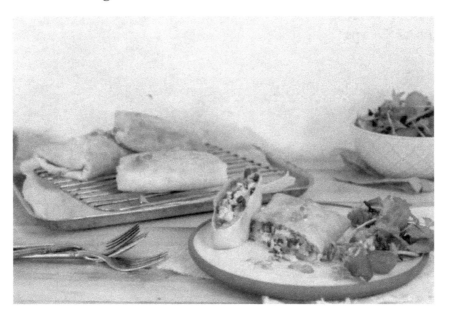

Method:

1. Heat oil on medium temperature in an air fryer. Cook capsicum for about five minutes until it starts to soften. Add mushrooms and cook them for another five mins until mushrooms become golden and evaporating any water left in the pan. Move mushrooms to another bowl. Leave them to cool for 10 mins.

2. Take a heatproof bowl and put spinach in it. Cover it with boiling water. Wait for 1 min until slightly wilted. Drain water and leave it to cool for about 10 mins.

3. Excessive spinach moisture is squeezed and applied to the capsicum mixture. Add the oregano, basil, ham and fetta. Season it with both salt & pepper. Mix it well to combine properly.

4. Put one wrapper on the smooth surface. Add 1 tbsp of tomato paste to the middle of the wrap. Cover it with a combination of 1-quarter of the capsicum. Roll up the wrap to completely enclose the filling, give it as the shape of parcel and folding the sides. To build four parcels, repeat the procedure with the remaining wraps, mixture of capsicum & tomato paste. Use oil spray on the tops.

5. Pre-heat the air fryer at 180 C temperature. Cook the parcels for 6 - 8 mins until they become golden & crispy, take out them and move to 2 more batches. Serve along with the salad.

60. Air Fryer Popcorn Fetta with Maple Hot Sauce

Ingredients:

- Marinated Fetta cubes - 265g
- Cajun for seasoning - 2 tsp.
- Breadcrumbs - 2/3 cups
- Corn flour - 2 tbsp.
- Egg - 1
- Chopped Fresh Coriander - 1 tbsp.
- Coriander leaves - for serving

Maple hot sauce:

- Maple syrup - 2 tbsp.
- Sriracha - 1 tbsps.

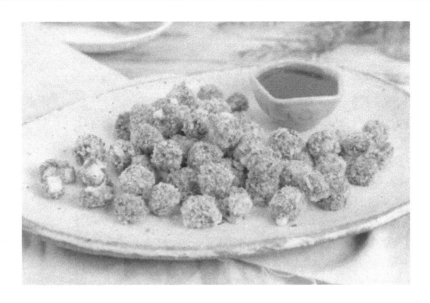

Method:

1. Drain the fetta, then reserve 1 tbsp of oil making sauce.

2. Take a bowl, mix the cornflour and the Cajun seasoning together. Beat the egg in another bowl. Take one more bowl and combine the breadcrumbs & cilantro in it. Season it with salt & pepper. Work in batches, coat the fetta in cornflour mixture, then dip in the egg. After that, toss them in breadcrumb mixture for coating. Place them on the plate and freeze them for one hour.

3. Take a saucepan, add Sriracha, reserved oil and maple syrup together and put on medium low heat. Stir it for 3 - 4 minutes continuously until sauce get start to thicken. Then, remove the maple sauce from heat.

4. Pre-heat the air fryer at 180C. Place the cubes of fetta in a single layer in the air fryer's pot. Cook them for 3 - 4 mins until just staring softened, and fettas become golden. Sprinkled with extra coriander leaves and serve them with the maple hot sauce.

61. Air fryer Steak Fajitas

Ingredients:

- Chopped tomatoes - 2 large
- Minced Jalapeno pepper - 1
- Cumin - 2 tsp.
- Lime juice - 1/4 cup
- Fresh minced Cilantro - 3 tbsp.
- Diced Red Onion - 1/2 cup
- 8-inches long Whole-wheat tortillas - 6

- Large onion - 1 sliced
- Salt - 3/4 tsp divided
- Beef steak - 1

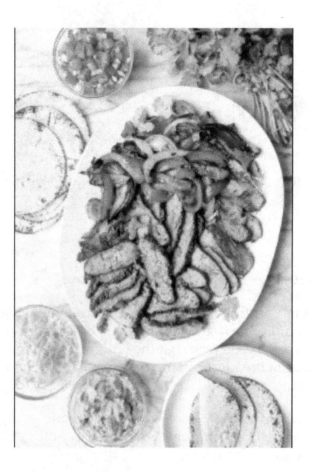

Method:

1. Mix first 5 ingredients in a clean bowl then stir in cumin and salt. Let it stand till before you serve.

2. Pre-heat the air fryer at 400 degrees. Sprinkle the cumin and salt with the steak that remain. Place them on buttered air-fryer pot and cook the steak until the meat reaches the appropriate thickness (a thermometer should read 135 ° for medium-rare; 140 °; moderate, 145 °), for 6 to 8 mins per side. Remove from the air fryer and leave for five min to stand.

3. Then, put the onion in the air-fryer pot. Cook it until get crispy-tender, stirring once for 2 - 3 mins. Thinly slice the steak and serve with onion & salsa in the tortillas. Serve it with avocado & lime slices if needed.

62. Air-Fryer Fajita-Stuffed Chicken

Ingredients:

- Boneless Chicken breast - 4
- Finely Sliced Onion - 1 small
- Finely Sliced Green pepper - 1/2 medium-sized
- Olive oil - 1 tbsp.
- Salt - 1/2 tsp.
- Chilli Powder - 1 tbsp.
- Cheddar Cheese - 4 ounces
- Cumin - 1 tsp.
- Salsa or jalapeno slices - optional

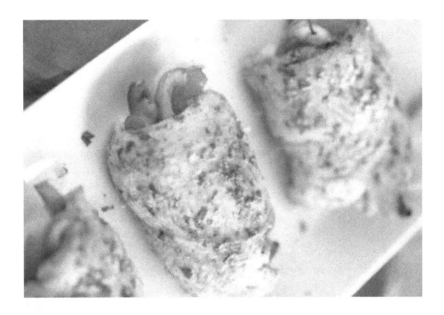

Method:

1. Pre-heat the air fryer at the 375 degrees. In the widest part of every chicken breast, cut a gap horizontally. Fill it with green pepper and onion. Combine olive oil and the seasonings in a clean bowl and apply over the chicken.

2. Place the chicken on a greased dish in the form of batches in an air-fryer pot. Cook it for 6 minutes. Stuff the chicken with cheese slices and secure the chicken pieces with toothpicks. Cook at 165° until for 6 to 8 minutes. Take off the toothpicks. Serve the delicious chicken with toppings of your choosing, if wanted.

63. Nashvilla Hot Chicken in an Air Fryer

Ingredients:

- Chicken Tenderloins - 2 pounds
- Plain flour - 1 cup
- Hot pepper Sauce - 2 tbsp.
- Egg - 1 large
- Salt - 1 tsp.
- Pepper - 1/2 tsp.
- Buttermilk - 1/2 cup
- Cayenne Pepper - 2 tbsp.
- Chilli powder - 1 tsp.
- Pickle Juice - 2 tbsp.
- Garlic Powder - 1/2 tsp.
- Paprika - 1 tsp.
- Brown Sugar - 2 tbsp.
- Olive oil - 1/2 cup
- Cooling oil for spray

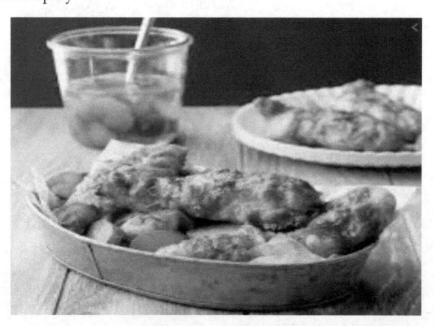

Method:

1. Combine pickle juice, hot sauce and salt in a clean bowl and coat the chicken on its both sides. Put it in the fridge, cover it, for a minimum 1 hour. Throwing away some marinade.

2. Pre-heat the air fryer at 375 degrees. Mix the flour, the remaining salt and the pepper in another bowl. Whisk together the buttermilk, eggs, pickle juice and hot sauce well. For coating the both sides, dip the chicken in plain flour; drip off the excess. Dip chicken in egg mixture and then again dip in flour mixture.

3. Arrange the single layer of chicken on a greased air-fryer pot and spray with cooking oil. Cook for 5 to 6 minutes until it becomes golden brown. Turn and spray well. Again, cook it until golden brown, for more 5-6 minutes.

4. Mix oil, brown sugar, cayenne pepper and seasonings together. Then, pour on the hot chicken and toss to cover. Serve the hot chicken with pickles.

64. Southern-style Chicken

Ingredients:

- Crushed Crackers - 2 cups (about 50)
- Fresh minced parsley - 1 tbsp.
- Paprika - 1 tsp.
- Pepper - 1/2 tsp.
- Garlic salt - 1 tsp.
- Fryer Chicken - 1
- Cumin - 1/4 tsp.
- Egg - 1
- Cooking Oil for spray

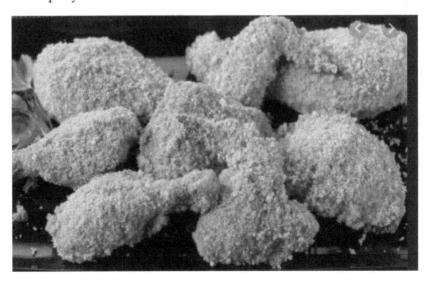

Method:

1. Set the temperature of an air fryer at 375 degrees. Mix the first 7 ingredients in a deep bowl. Beat an egg in deep bowl. Soak the chicken in egg, then pat in the cracker mixture for proper coat. Place the chicken in a single layer on the greased air-fryer pot and spray with cooking oil.

2. Cook it for 10 minutes. Change the sides of chicken and squirt with cooking oil spray. Cook until the chicken becomes golden brown & juices seem to be clear, for 10 - 20 minutes longer.

65. Chicken Parmesan in an Air Fryer

Ingredients:

- Breadcrumbs - 1/2 cup
- Pepper - 1/4 tsp.
- Pasta Sauce - 1 cup
- Boneless Chicken breast - 4
- Mozzarella Cheese - 1 cup
- Parmesan Cheese - 1/3 cup
- Large Eggs - 2
- Fresh basil - Optional

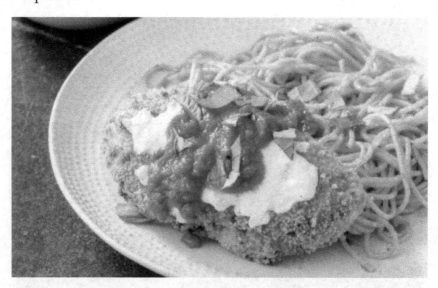

Method:

1. Set the temperature of an air-fryer at 375 degrees. In a deep bowl, beat the eggs gently. Combine the breadcrumbs, pepper and parmesan cheese in another bowl. Dip the chicken in beaten egg and coat the chicken parmesan with breadcrumbs mixture.

2. In an air-fryer pot, put the chicken in single layer. Cook the chicken for 10 to 12 mins with changing the sides partially. Cover the chicken with cheese and sauce. Cook it for 3 to 4 minutes until cheese has melted. Then, sprinkle with basil leaves and serve.

66. Lemon Chicken Thigh in an Air Fryer

Ingredients:

- Bone-in Chicken thighs- 4
- Pepper - 1/8 tsp.
- Salt - 1/8 tsp.
- Pasta Sauce - 1 cup
- Lemon Juice - 1 tbsp.
- Lemon Zest - 1 tsp.
- Minced Garlic - 3 cloves
- Butter - 1/4 cup
- Dried or Fresh Rosemary - 1 tsp.
- Dried or Fresh Thyme - 1/4 tsp.

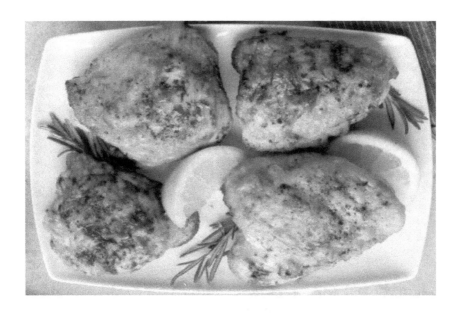

Method:

1.   Pre-heat   the   air fryer   at 400   degrees.   Combine   the   butter, thyme, rosemary, garlic, lemon juice & zest in a clean bowl. Spread a mixture on each of the thigh's skin. Use salt and pepper to sprinkle.

2. Place the chicken, then side up the skin, in a greased air-fryer pot. Cook for 20 mins and flip once. Switch the chicken again (side up the skin) and cook it for about 5 mins until the thermometer will read 170 degrees to 175 degrees. Then, place in the serving plate and serve it.

67. Salmon with Maple-Dijon Glaze in air fryer

Ingredients:

- Salmon Fillets - 4 (about ounces)
- Salt - 1/4 tsp.
- Pepper - 1/4 tsp.
- Butter - 3 tbsp.
- Mustard - 1 tbsp.
- Lemon Juice - 1 medium-sized
- Garlic clove - 1 minced
- Olive oil

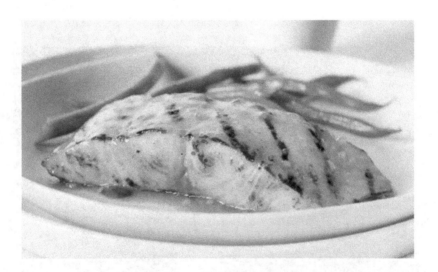

Method:

1. Pre-heat the air fryer at 400 degrees. Melt butter in a medium-sized pan on medium temperature. Put the mustard, minced garlic, maple syrup & lemon juice. Lower the heat and cook for 2 - 3 minutes before the mixture thickens significantly. Take off from the heat and set aside for few mins.

2. Brush the salmon with olive oil and also sprinkle the salt and pepper on it.

3. In an air fryer bucket, put the fish in a single baking sheet. Cook for 5 to 7 mins until fish is browned and easy to flake rapidly with help of fork. Sprinkle before to serve the salmon with sauce.

68. Air Fryer Roasted Beans

Ingredients:

- Fresh Sliced Mushrooms - 1/2 pounds
- Green Beans cut into 2-inch wedges - 1 pound
- Italian Seasoning - 1 tsp.
- Pepper - 1/8 tsp.
- Salt - 1/4 tsp.
- Red onion - 1 small
- Olive oil - 2 tbsp.

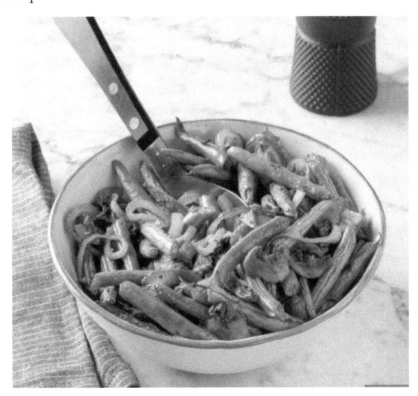

Method:

1. Pre-heat the air fryer at 375 degrees. Merge all of the ingredients in the large-sized bowl by tossing.

2. Assemble the vegetables on the greased air-fryer pot. Cook for 8 -10 minutes until become tender. Redistribute by tossing and cook for 8-10 minutes until they get browned.

69. Air Fried Radishes

Ingredients:

- Quartered Radishes - (about 6 cups)
- Fresh Oregano - 1 tbsp.
- Dried Oregano - 1 tbsp.
- Pepper - 1/8 tsp.
- Salt - 1/4 tsp.
- Olive Oil - 3 tbsp.

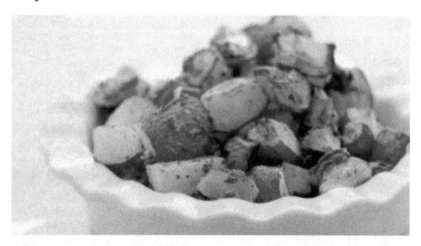

Method:

1. Set the temperature of an air fryer to 375 degrees. Mix the rest of the ingredients with radishes. In an air-fryer pot, put the radishes on greased dish.

2. Cook them for 12-15 minutes until they become crispy & tender with periodically stirring. Take out from the air fryer and serve the radishes in a clean dish.

70. Air Fried Catfish Nuggets

Ingredients

- Catfish fillets (1 inch) - 1 pound
- Seasoned fish fry coating - 3/4 cup
- Cooking oil - to spray

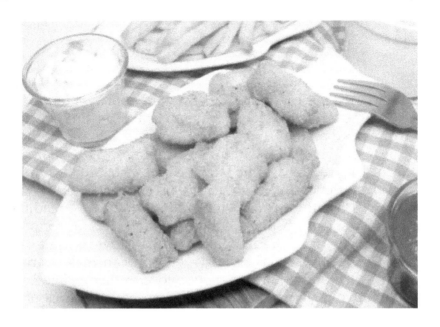

Method

1. Set the temperature of an air fryer to 200C.

2. Coat catfish pieces with seasoned coating mix by proper mixing from all sides.

3. Place nuggets evenly in an oiled air fryer pot. Spray both sides of nuggets with cooking oil. You can work in batches if the size of your air fryer is small.

4. Air fry nuggets for 5-8 minutes. Change sides of nuggets with the help of tongs and cook for more 5 minutes. Shift these delicious nuggets in a clean plate and serve immediately.

CONCLUSION:

This manual served you the easiest, quick, healthy and delicious foods that are made in an air fryer. It is also very necessary to cook food easily and timely without getting so much tired. We've discussed all the 70 easy, short, quick, delicious and healthy foods and dishes. These recipes can be made within few minutes. This manual provides the handiest or helpful cooking recipes for the busy people who are performing their routine tasks. Instead of ordering the costly or unhealthy food from hotels, you will be able to make the easy, tasty and healthy dishes with minimum cost. By reading this the most informative handbook, you can learn, experience or make lots of recipes in an air with great taste because cooking food traditionally on the stove is quite difficult for the professional persons. With the help of an air fryer, you can make various dishes for a single person as well as the entire family timely and effortlessly. We conclude that this cook book will maintain your health and it would also be the source of enjoying dishes without doing great effort in less and budget.

Vegan Air Fryer Cookbook

Cook and Taste 50+ High-Protein Recipes. Kickstart Muscles and Body Transformation, Kill Hunger and Feel More Energetic

By

Chef Mirco Miccio

Table of Contents

Introduction

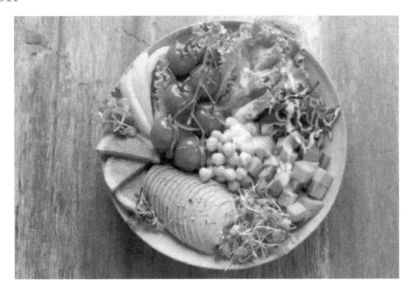

To have a good, satisfying life, a balanced diet is important. Tiredness and susceptibility to illnesses, many severe, arise from a lifestyle so full of junk food. Our community, sadly, does not neglect unsafe choices. People turn to immoral practices in order to satisfy desire, leading to animal torture. Two of the key explanations that people adhere to vegetarianism, a vegan-based diet that often excludes animal foods such as cheese, beef, jelly, and honey, are fitness and animal welfare.

It's essential for vegetarians to get the most nutrients out of any food, and that's where frying using an air fryer shines. The air fryer cooking will maintain as many nutrients as possible from beans and veggies, and the gadget makes it incredibly simple to cook nutritious food.

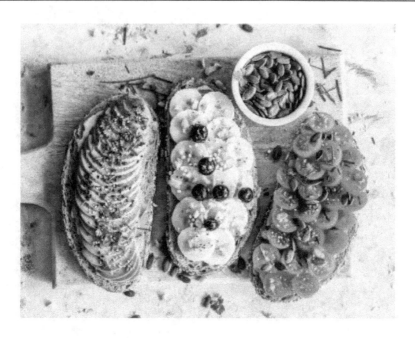

Although there are prepared vegan alternatives, the healthier choice, and far less pricey, is still to prepare your own recipes. This book provides the very first moves to being a vegan and offers 50 quick breakfast recipes, sides, snacks, and much more, so you have a solid base on which to develop.

This book will teach you all you need to thrive, whether you are either a vegan and only need more meal choices or have just begun contemplating transforming your diet.

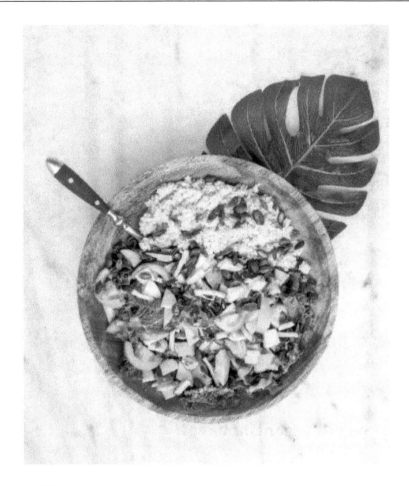

What is Cooking Vegan?

In recent decades, vegetarianism has become quite common, as individuals understand just how toxic the eating patterns of civilization have become. We are a society that enjoys meat, and, unfortunately, we go to dishonest measures to get the food we like. More citizens are choosing to give up beef and, unlike vegans, other livestock items due to various health issues, ethical issues, or both. Their diet moves to one focused on plants, whole grains, beans, fruit, seeds, nuts, and vegan varieties of the common dish.

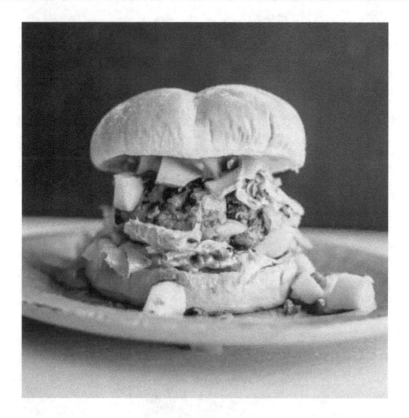

What advantages would veganism have?

There are a lot of advantages to a diet away from all animal items. Only a few includes:

- Healthier hair, skin, and nails

- High energy

- Fewer chances of flu and cold

- Fewer migraines

- Increased tolerance to cancer

- Strengthened fitness of the heart

Although research has proven that veganism will contribute to reducing BMI, it must not be followed for the mere sake of weight reduction. "Vegan" does not indicate "lower-calorie," and if you wish to reduce weight, other healthier activities, including exercising and consuming water, can complement the diet.

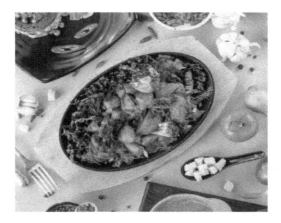

Air Fryer

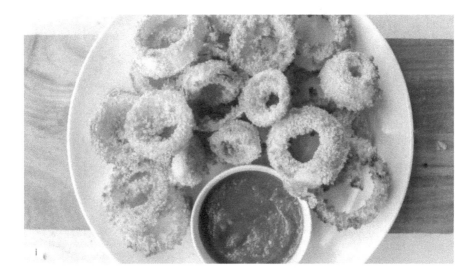

A common kitchen gadget used to create fried foods such as beef, baked goods and potato chips is an air fryer. It provides a crunchy, crisp coating by blowing hot air across the food. This also leads to a chemical reaction commonly known as the Maillard effect, which happens in the presence of heat in between reducing sugar and amino acid. This adds to shifts in food color and taste. Due to the reduced amount of calories and fat, air-fried items are marketed as a healthier substitute to deep-fried foods.

Rather than fully soaking the food in fat, air-frying utilizes just a teaspoon to create a flavor and feel equivalent to deep-fried foods.

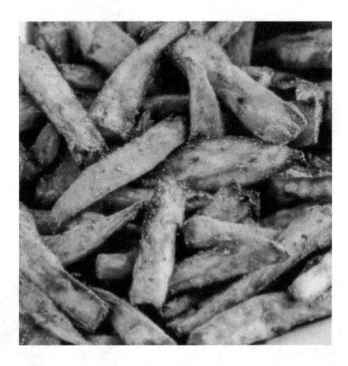

The flavor and appearance of the fried food in the air are similar to the deep fryer outcomes: On the surface, crispy; from the inside, soft. You do need to use a limited amount of oil, though, or any at all (based on what you're baking). But indeed, contrary to deep frying, if you agree to use only 1-2 teaspoons of plant-based oil with spices and you stuck to air-frying vegetables rather than anything else, air frying is certainly a better option.

The secret to weight loss, decreased likelihood of cardiovascular illness and better long-term wellbeing as we mature is any gadget that assists you and your friends in your vegetarian game.

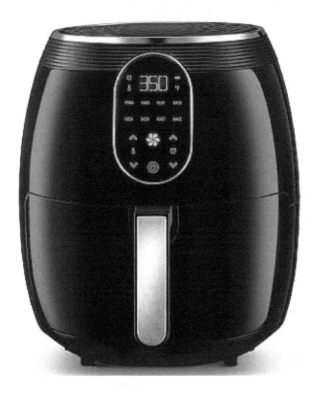

Air fryer's Working Process:

The air fryer is a worktop kitchen gadget that operates in the same manner as a traditional oven. To become acquainted with the operating theory of the traditional oven, you will need a little study. The air fryer uses rotating hot air to fry and crisp your meal, close to the convection oven. In a traditional convection oven, the airflow relies on revolving fans, which blast hot air around to produce an even or equalized temperature dispersal throughout the oven.

This is compared to the upward airflow of standard ovens, where the warm place is typically the oven's tip. And although the air fryer is not quite like the convection oven, it is a great approximation of it in the field of airflow for most components. The gadget has an air inlet at the top that lets air in and a hot air outlet at the side. All of these features are used to monitor the temperature within the air fryer. Temperatures will rise to 230 ° C, based on the sort of air fryer you're buying.

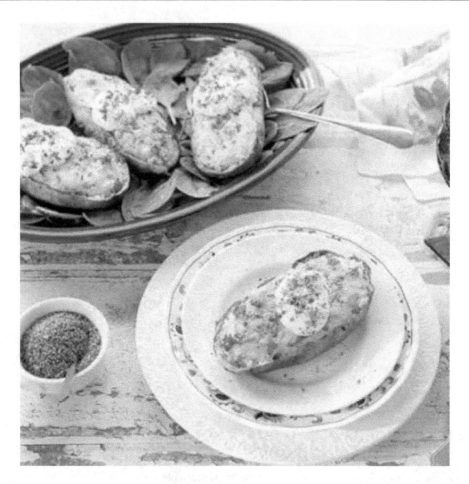

In conjunction with any grease, this hot air is used for cooking the food in the bowl within the device, if you like. Yes, if you want a taste of the oil, you should apply more oil. To jazz up the taste of the meal, simply add a little more to the blend. But the key concept behind the air fryer is to reduce the consumption of calories and fat without reducing the amount of taste.

Using air frying rather than deep frying saves between 70-80 calories, according to researchers. The growing success of recipes for air fryers is simply attributed to its impressive performance. It is simple to use and less time-consuming than conventional ovens.

This is more or less a lottery win for people searching for healthy alternative to deep-frying, as demonstrated by its widespread popularity in many homes today. In contrast to conventional ovens or deep frying, the air fryer creates crispy, crunchy, wonderful, and far fewer fatty foods in less duration. For certain individuals like us; this is what distinguishes air fryer recipes.

Tips for using an Air Fryer

1. The food is cooked easily. Air fried, unlike conventional cooking techniques, cut the cooking time a great deal. Therefore, to stop burning the food or getting a not-so-great flavor, it is best to hold a close eye on the gadget. Notice, remember that the smaller the food on the basket, the shorter the cooking period, which implies that the food cooks quicker.

2. You may need to reduce the temperature at first. Bear in mind that air fryers depend on the flow of hot air, which heats up rapidly. This ensures that it's better, to begin with, a low temperature so that the food cooks equally. It is likely that when the inside is already cooking, the exterior of the food is all cooked and begins to become dark or too dry.

3. When air fryers are in operation, they create some noise. If you are new to recipes for air fryers, you may have to realize that air fryers create noise while working. When it's in service, a whirring tone emanates from the device. However, the slight annoyance pales in contrast to the various advantages of having an air fryer.

4. Hold the grate within the container at all hours. As previously mentioned, the air fryer has a container inside it, where the food is put and permitted to cook. This helps hot air to flow freely around the food, allowing for even cooking.

5. Don't stuff the air fryer with so much food at once. If you plan to make a meal for one guy, with only one batch, you would most definitely be able to get your cooking right. If you're cooking for two or more individuals, you can need to plan the food in groups. With a 4 - 5 quart air fryer, you can always need to cook in groups, depending on the size and sort of air fryer you have. This not only means that your device works longer but also

keeps your food from cooking unevenly. You shouldn't have to turn the air fryer off as you pull out the basket since it simply turns off on its own until the basket is out. Often, make sure the drawer is completely retracted; otherwise, the fryer would not turn back on.

6. Take the basket out of the mix and mix the ingredients. You might need to move the food around or switch it over once every few minutes, based on the dish you're preparing and the time it takes to prepare your dinner.

The explanation for this is that even cooking can be done. Certain recipes involve the foods in the basket to shake and shuffle throughout the cooking phase. And an easy-to-understand checklist is given for each recipe to direct you thru the cycle.

7. The air fryer does not need cooking mist. It isn't needed. In order to prevent the urge to use non-stick frying spray in the container, you must deliberately take care of this. The basket is now coated with a non-stick covering, so what you need to do is fill your meal inside the container and push it back in.

Outcome

You can create nutritious meals very simply and fast, right in the comfort of your house. There are many excellent recipes for producing healthier meals and nutritious foods, which you can notice in the air fryer recipes illustrated in this book. However, you'll need to pay careful attention to the ingredients and know-how to easily use the air fryer to do this. To get straightforward guidance on installation and usage, you can need to refer to the company's manual.

CHAPTER 1: Breakfast Recipes

1. Toasted French toast

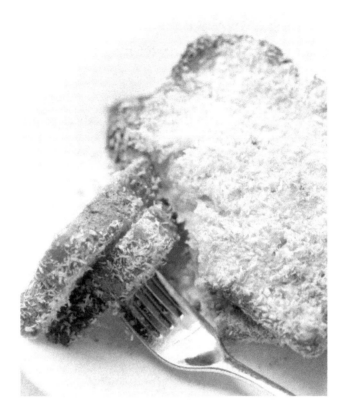

Preparation time: 2 minutes

Cooking time: 5 minutes

Servings: 1 people

Ingredients:

- ½ Cup of Unsweetened Shredded Coconut

- 1 Tsp. Baking Powder

- ½ Cup Lite Culinary Coconut Milk

- 2 Slices of Gluten-Free Bread (use your favorite)

Directions:

1. Stir together the baking powder and coconut milk in a large rimmed pot.

2. On a tray, layout your ground coconut.

3. Pick each loaf of your bread and dip it in your coconut milk for the very first time, and then pass it to the ground coconut, let it sit for a few minutes, then cover the slice entirely with the coconut.

4. Place the covered bread loaves in your air fryer, cover it, adjust the temperature to about 350 ° F and set the clock for around 4 minutes.

5. Take out from your air fryer until done, and finish with some maple syrup of your choice. French toast is done. Enjoy!

2. Vegan Casserole

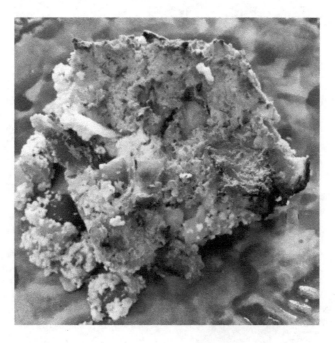

Preparation time: 10-12 minutes

Cooking time: 15-20 minutes

Servings: 2-3 people

Ingredients:

- 1/2 cup of cooked quinoa

- 1 tbsp. of lemon juice

- 2 tbsp. of water

- 2 tbsp. of plain soy yogurt

- 2 tbsp. of nutritional yeast

- 7 ounces of extra-firm tofu about half a block, drained but not pressed

- 1/2 tsp. of ground cumin

- 1/2 tsp. of red pepper flakes

- 1/2 tsp. of freeze-dried dill

- 1/2 tsp. of black pepper

- 1/2 tsp. of salt

- 1 tsp. of dried oregano

- 1/2 cup of diced shiitake mushrooms

- 1/2 cup of diced bell pepper I used a combination of red and green

- 2 small celery stalks chopped

- 1 large carrot chopped

- 1 tsp. of minced garlic

- 1 small onion diced

- 1 tsp. of olive oil

Directions:

1. Warm the olive oil over medium-low heat in a big skillet. Add your onion and garlic and simmer till the onion is transparent (for about 3 to 6 minutes). Add your

bell pepper, carrot, and celery and simmer for another 3 minutes. Mix the oregano, mushrooms, pepper, salt, cumin, dill, and red pepper powder. Mix completely and lower the heat to low. If the vegetables tend to cling, stir regularly and add in about a teaspoon of water.

2. Pulse the nutritional yeast, tofu, water, yogurt, and some lemon juice in a food mixer until fluffy. To your skillet, add your tofu mixture. Add in half a cup of cooked quinoa. Mix thoroughly.

3. Move to a microwave-proof plate or tray that works for your air fryer basket.

4. Cook for around 15 minutes at about 350°F (or 18 to 20 minutes at about 330°F, till it turns golden brown).

5. Please take out your plate or tray from your air fryer and let it rest for at least five minutes before eating.

3. Vegan Omelet

Preparation time: 15 minutes

Cooking time: 16 minutes

Servings: 3 people

Ingredients:

- ½ cup of grated vegan cheese

- 1 tbsp. of water

- 1 tbsp. of brags

- 3 tbsp. of nutritional yeast

- ¼ tsp. of basil

- ¼ tsp. of garlic powder

- ¼ tsp. of onion powder

- ¼ tsp. of pepper

- ½ tsp. of cumin

- ½ tsp. of turmeric

- ¼ tsp. of salt

- ¼ cup of chickpea flour (or you may use any bean flour)

- ½ cup of finely diced veggies (like chard, kale, dried mushrooms, spinach, watermelon radish etc.)

- half a piece of tofu (organic high in protein kind)

Directions:

4. Blend all your ingredients in a food blender or mixer, excluding the vegetables and cheese.

5. Move the batter from the blender to a container and combine the vegetables and cheese in it. Since it's faster, you could use both hands to combine it.

6. Brush the base of your air fryer bucket with some oil.

7. Put a couple of parchment papers on your counter. On the top of your parchment paper, place a cookie cutter of your desire.

8. In your cookie cutter, push 1/6 of the paste. Then raise and put the cookie cutter on a different section of your parchment paper.

9. Redo the process till you have about 6 pieces using the remainder of the paste.

10. Put 2 or 3 of your omelets at the base of your air fryer container. Using some oil, brush the topsides of the omelets.

11. Cook for around 5 minutes at about 370 °, turn and bake for another 4 minutes or more if needed. And redo with the omelets that remain.

12. Offer with sriracha mayo or whatever kind of dipping sauce you prefer. Or use them for a sandwich at breakfast.

4. Waffles with Vegan chicken

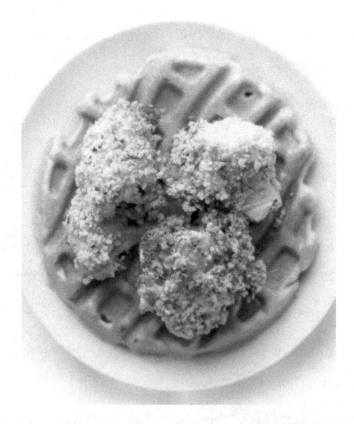

Preparation time: 10 minutes

Cooking time: 15 minutes

Servings: 2 people

Ingredients:

Fried Vegan Chicken:

- ¼ to ½ teaspoon of Black Pepper

- ½ teaspoon of Paprika

- ½ teaspoon of Onion Powder

- ½ teaspoon of Garlic Powder

- 2 teaspoon of Dried Parsley

- 2 Cups of Gluten-Free Panko

- ¼ Cup of Cornstarch

- 1 Cup of Unsweetened Non-Dairy Milk

- 1 Small Head of Cauliflower

Yummy Cornmeal Waffles:

- ½ teaspoon of Pure Vanilla Extract

- ¼ Cup of Unsweetened Applesauce

- ½ Cup of Unsweetened Non-Dairy Milk

- 1 to 2 TB Erythritol (or preferred sweetener)

- 1 teaspoon Baking Powder

- ¼ Cup of Stoneground Cornmeal

- ⅔ Cup of Gluten-Free All-Purpose Flour

Toppings:

- Vegan Butter

- Hot Sauce

- Pure Maple Syrup

Directions:

For making your Vegan Fried Chicken:

1. Dice the cauliflower (you wouldn't have to be careful in this) into big florets and put it aside.

2. Mix the cornstarch and milk in a tiny pot.

3. Throw the herbs, panko, and spices together in a big bowl or dish.

4. In the thick milk mixture, soak your cauliflower florets, then cover the soaked bits in the prepared panko mix before putting the wrapped floret into your air fryer bucket.

5. For the remaining of your cauliflower, redo the same process.

6. Set your air fryer clock for around 15 minutes to about 400 ° F and let the cauliflower air fry.

For making you're Waffles:

1. Oil a regular waffle iron and warm it up.

2. Mix all your dry ingredients in a pot, and then blend in your wet ingredients until you have a thick mixture.

3. To create a big waffle, utilize ½ of the mixture and redo the process to create another waffle for a maximum of two persons.

To Organize:

1. Put on dishes your waffles, place each with ½ of the cooked cauliflower, now drizzle with the hot sauce, syrup, and any extra toppings that you want. Serve warm!

5. Tempeh Bacon

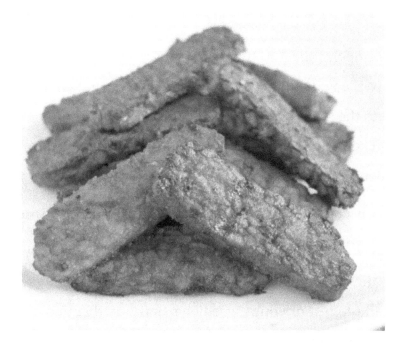

Preparation time: 15 minutes plus 2 hour marinating time

Cooking time: 10 minutes

Servings: 4 people

Ingredients:

- ½ teaspoon of freshly grated black pepper

- ½ teaspoon of onion powder

- ½ teaspoon of garlic powder

- 1 ½ teaspoon of smoked paprika

- 1 teaspoon of apple cider vinegar

- 1 tablespoon of olive oil (plus some more for oiling your air fryer)

- 3 tablespoon of pure maple syrup

- ¼ cup of gluten-free, reduced-sodium tamari

- 8 oz. of gluten-free tempeh

Directions:

1. Break your Tempeh cube into two parts and boil for about 10 minutes, some more if required. To the rice cooker bowl, add a cup of warm water. Then, put the pieces of tempeh into the steamer basket of the unit. Close the cover, push the button for heat or steam cooking (based on your rice cooker's type or brand), and adjust the steaming timer for around 10 minutes.

2. Let the tempeh cool completely before taking it out of the rice cooker or your steamer basket for around 5 minutes.

3. Now make the sauce while cooking the tempeh. In a 9" x 13" baking tray, incorporate all the rest of your ingredients and mix them using a fork. Then set it aside and ready the tempeh.

4. Put the tempeh steamed before and cooled on a chopping board, and slice into strips around 1/4' wide. Put each slice gently in the sauce. Then roll over each slice gently. Seal and put in the fridge for two to three hours or even overnight, rotating once or twice during the time.

5. Turn the bits gently one more time until you are about to create the tempeh bacon. And if you would like, you may spoon over any leftover sauce.

6. Put your crisper plate/tray into the air fryer if yours came with one instead of a built-in one. Oil the base of your crisper tray or your air fryer basket slightly with some olive oil or using an olive oil spray that is anti-aerosol.

7. Put the tempeh slices in a thin layer gently in your air fryer bucket. If you have a tiny air fryer, you will have to air fry it in two or multiple rounds. Air fry for around 10-15 minutes at about 325 ° F before the slices are lightly golden but not

burnt. You may detach your air fryer container to inspect it and make sure it's not burnt. It normally takes about 10 minutes.

6. Delicious Potato Pancakes

Preparation time: 5 minutes

Cooking time: 15 minutes

Servings: 4 people

Ingredients:

- black pepper according to taste

- 3 tablespoon of flour

- ¼ teaspoon of pepper

- ¼ teaspoon of salt

- ½ teaspoon of garlic powder

- 2 tablespoon of unsalted butter

- ¼ cup of milk

- 1 beaten egg

- 1 medium onion, chopped

Directions:

1. Preheat the fryer to about 390° F and combine the potatoes, garlic powder, eggs, milk, onion, pepper, butter, and salt in a small bowl; add in the flour and make a batter.

2. Shape around 1/4 cup of your batter into a cake.

3. In the fryer's cooking basket, put the cakes and cook for a couple of minutes.

4. Serve and enjoy your treat!

CHAPTER 2: Air Fryer Main Dishes

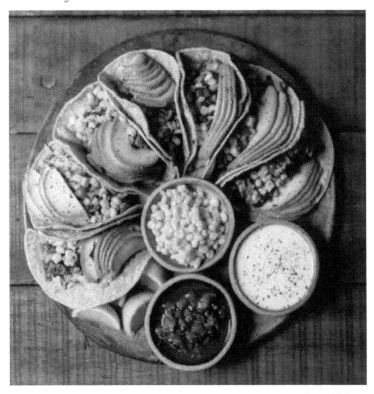

1. Mushroom 'n Bell Pepper Pizza

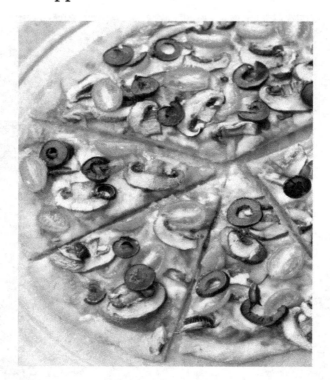

Preparation time: 5 minutes

Cooking time: 10 minutes

Servings: 10 people

Ingredients:

- salt and pepper according to taste

- 2 tbsp. of parsley

- 1 vegan pizza dough

- 1 shallot, chopped

- 1 cup of oyster mushrooms, chopped

- ¼ red bell pepper, chopped

Directions:

1. Preheat your air fryer to about 400°F.

2. Cut the pie dough into small squares. Just set them aside.

3. Put your bell pepper, shallot, oyster mushroom, and parsley all together into a mixing dish.

4. According to taste, sprinkle with some pepper and salt.

5. On top of your pizza cubes, put your topping.

6. Put your pizza cubes into your air fryer and cook for about 10 minutes.

2. Veggies Stuffed Eggplants

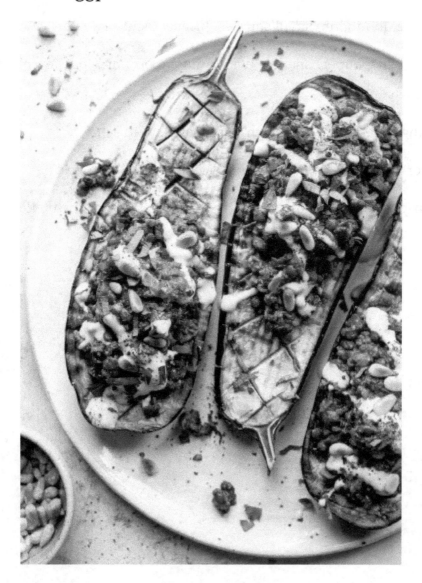

Preparation time: 5 minutes

Cooking time: 14 minutes

Servings: 5 people

Ingredients:

- 2 tbsp. of tomato paste

- Salt and ground black pepper, as required

- ½ tsp. of garlic, chopped

- 1 tbsp. of vegetable oil

- 1 tbsp. of fresh lime juice

- ½ green bell pepper, seeded and chopped

- ¼ cup of cottage cheese, chopped

- 1 tomato, chopped

- 1 onion, chopped

- 10 small eggplants, halved lengthwise

Directions:

1. Preheat your air fryer to about 320°F and oil the container of your air fryer.

2. Cut a strip longitudinally from all sides of your eggplant and scrape out the pulp in a medium-sized bowl.

3. Add lime juice on top of your eggplants and place them in the container of your Air Fryer.

4. Cook for around a couple of minutes and extract from your Air Fryer.

5. Heat the vegetable oil on medium-high heat in a pan and add the onion and garlic.

6. Sauté for around 2 minutes and mix in the tomato, salt, eggplant flesh, and black pepper.

7. Sauté and add bell pepper, tomato paste, cheese, and cilantro for roughly 3 minutes.

8. Cook for around a minute and put this paste into your eggplants.

9. Shut each eggplant with its lids and adjust the Air Fryer to 360°F.

10. Organize and bake for around 5 minutes in your Air Fryer Basket.

11. Dish out on a serving tray and eat hot.

3. Air-fried Falafel

Preparation time: 10 minutes

Cooking time: 25 minutes

Servings: 6 people

Ingredients:

- Salt and black pepper according to taste

- 1 teaspoon of chili powder

- 2 teaspoon of ground coriander

- 2 teaspoon of ground cumin

- 1 onion, chopped

- 4 garlic cloves, chopped

- Juice of 1 lemon

- 1 cup of fresh parsley, chopped

- ½ cup of chickpea flour

Directions:

1. Add flour, coriander, chickpeas, lemon juice, parsley, onion, garlic, chili, cumin, salt, turmeric, and pepper to a processor and mix until mixed, not too battery; several chunks should be present.

2. Morph the paste into spheres and hand-press them to ensure that they are still around.

3. Spray using some spray oil and place them in a paper-lined air fryer bucket; if necessary, perform in groups.

4. Cook for about 14 minutes at around 360°F, rotating once mid-way through the cooking process.

5. They must be light brown and crispy.

4. Almond Flour Battered Wings

Preparation time: 10 minutes

Cooking time: 25 minutes

Servings: 4 people

Ingredients:

- Salt and pepper according to taste

- 4 tbsp. of minced garlic

- 2 tbsp. of stevia powder

- 16 pieces of vegan chicken wings

- ¾ cup of almond flour

- ¼ cup of butter, melted

Directions:

1. Preheat your air fryer for about 5 minutes.

2. Mix the stevia powder, almond flour, vegan chicken wings, and garlic in a mixing dish. According to taste, sprinkle with some black pepper and salt.

3. Please put it in the bucket of your air fryer and cook at about 400°F for around 25 minutes.

4. Ensure you give your fryer container a shake midway through the cooking process.

5. Put in a serving dish after cooking and add some melted butter on top. Toss it to coat it completely.

5. Spicy Tofu

Preparation time: 5 minutes

Cooking time: 13 minutes

Servings: 3 people

Ingredients:

- Salt and black pepper, according to taste

- 1 tsp. of garlic powder

- 1 tsp. of onion powder

- 1½ tsp. of paprika

- 1½ tbsp. of avocado oil

- 3 tsp. of cornstarch

- 1 (14-ounces) block extra-firm tofu, pressed and cut into ¾-inch cubes

Directions:

1. Preheat your air fryer to about 390°F and oil the container of your air fryer with some spray oil.

2. In a medium-sized bowl, blend the cornstarch, oil, tofu, and spices and mix to cover properly.

3. In the Air Fryer basket, place the tofu bits and cook for around a minute, flipping twice between the cooking times.

4. On a serving dish, spread out the tofu and enjoy it warm.

6. Sautéed Bacon with Spinach

Preparation time: 5 minutes

Cooking time: 9 minutes

Servings: 2 people

Ingredients:

- 1 garlic clove, minced

- 2 tbsp. of olive oil

- 4-ounce of fresh spinach

- 1 onion, chopped

- 3 meatless bacon slices, chopped

Directions:

1. Preheat your air fryer at about 340° F and oil the air fryer's tray with some olive oil or cooking oil spray.

2. In the Air Fryer basket, put garlic and olive oil.

3. Cook and add in the onions and bacon for around 2 minutes.

4. Cook and mix in the spinach for approximately 3 minutes.

5. Cook for 4 more minutes and plate out in a bowl to eat.

7. Garden Fresh Veggie Medley

Preparation time: 5 minutes

Cooking time: 15 minutes

Servings: 4 people

Ingredients:

- 1 tbsp. of balsamic vinegar

- 1 tbsp. of olive oil

- 2 tbsp. of herbs de Provence

- 2 garlic cloves, minced

- 2 small onions, chopped

- 3 tomatoes, chopped

- 1 zucchini, chopped

- 1 eggplant, chopped

- 2 yellow bell peppers seeded and chopped

- Salt and black pepper, according to taste.

Directions:

1. Preheat your air fryer at about 355° F and oil up the air fryer basket.

2. In a medium-sized bowl, add all the ingredients and toss to cover completely.

3. Move to the basket of your Air Fryer and cook for around 15 minutes.

4. After completing the cooking time, let it sit in the air fryer for around 5 minutes and plate out to serve warm.

8. Colorful Vegetable Croquettes

Preparation time: 5 minutes

Cooking time: 10 minutes

Servings: 4 people

Ingredients:

- 1/2 cup of parmesan cheese, grated

- 2 eggs

- 1/4 cup of coconut flour

- 1/2 cup of almond flour

- 2 tbsp. of olive oil

- 3 tbsp. of scallions, minced

- 1 clove garlic, minced

- 1 bell pepper, chopped

- 1/2 cup of mushrooms, chopped

- 1/2 tsp. of cayenne pepper

- Salt and black pepper, according to taste.

- 2 tbsp. of butter

- 4 tbsp. of milk

- 1/2 pound of broccoli

Directions:

1. Boil your broccoli in a medium-sized saucepan for up to around 20 minutes. With butter, milk, black pepper, salt, and cayenne pepper, rinse the broccoli and mash it.

2. Add in the bell pepper, mushrooms, garlic, scallions, and olive oil and blend properly. Form into patties with the blend.

3. Put the flour in a deep bowl; beat your eggs in a second bowl; then put the parmesan cheese in another bowl.

4. Dip each patty into your flour, accompanied by the eggs and lastly the parmesan cheese, push to hold the shape.

5. Cook for around 16 minutes, turning midway through the cooking period, in the preheated Air Fryer at about 370° F. Bon appétit!

9. Cheesy Mushrooms

Preparation time: 3 minutes

Cooking time: 8 minutes

Servings: 4 people

Ingredients:

- 1 tsp. of dried dill

- 2 tbsp. of Italian dried mixed herbs

- 2 tbsp. of olive oil

- 2 tbsp. of cheddar cheese, grated

- 2 tbsp. of mozzarella cheese, grated

- Salt and freshly ground black pepper, according to taste

- 6-ounce of button mushrooms stemmed

Directions:

Preheat the air fryer at around 355° F and oil your air fryer basket.

In a mixing bowl, combine the Italian dried mixed herbs, mushrooms, salt, oil, and black pepper and mix well to cover.

In the Air Fryer bucket, place the mushrooms and cover them with some cheddar cheese and mozzarella cheese.

To eat, cook for around 8 minutes and scatter with dried dill.

10. Greek-style Roasted Vegetables

Preparation time: 10 minutes

Cooking time: 25 minutes

Servings: 3 people

Ingredients:

- 1/2 cup of Kalamata olives, pitted

- 1 (28-ounce) canned diced tomatoes with juice

- 1/2 tsp. of dried basil

- Sea salt and freshly cracked black pepper, according to taste

- 1 tsp. of dried rosemary

- 1 cup of dry white wine

- 2 tbsp. of extra-virgin olive oil

- 2 bell peppers, cut into 1-inch chunks

- 1 red onion, sliced

- 1/2 pound of zucchini, cut into 1-inch chunks

- 1/2 pound of cauliflower, cut into 1-inch florets

- 1/2 pound of butternut squash, peeled and cut into 1-inch chunks

Directions:

1. Add some rosemary, wine, olive oil, black pepper, salt, and basil along with your vegetables toss until well-seasoned.

2. Onto a lightly oiled baking dish, add 1/2 of the canned chopped tomatoes; scatter to fill the base of your baking dish.

3. Add in the vegetables and add the leftover chopped tomatoes to the top. On top of tomatoes, spread the Kalamata olives.

4. Bake for around 20 minutes at about 390° F in the preheated Air Fryer, turning the dish midway through your cooking cycle. Serve it hot and enjoy it!

11. Vegetable Kabobs with Simple Peanut Sauce

Preparation time: 10 minutes

Cooking time: 30 minutes

Servings: 4 people

Ingredients:

- 1/3 tsp. of granulated garlic

- 1 tsp. of dried rosemary, crushed

- 1 tsp. of red pepper flakes, crushed

- Sea salt and ground black pepper, according to your taste.

- 2 tbsp. of extra-virgin olive oil

- 8 small button mushrooms, cleaned

- 8 pearl onions, halved

- 2 bell peppers, diced into 1-inch pieces

- 8 whole baby potatoes, diced into 1-inch pieces

Peanut Sauce:

- 1/2 tsp. of garlic salt

- 1 tbsp. of soy sauce

- 1 tbsp. of balsamic vinegar

- 2 tbsp. of peanut butter

Directions:

1. For a few minutes, dunk the wooden chopsticks in water.

2. String the vegetables onto your chopsticks; drip some olive oil all over your chopsticks with the vegetables on it; dust with seasoning.

3. Cook for about 1 minute at 400°F in the preheated Air Fryer.

Peanut Sauce:

1. In the meantime, mix the balsamic vinegar with some peanut butter, garlic salt and some soy sauce in a tiny dish. Offer the kabobs with a side of peanut sauce. Eat warm!

12. Hungarian Mushroom Pilaf

Preparation time: 10 minutes

Cooking time: 50 minutes

Servings: 4 people

Ingredients:

- 1 tsp. of sweet Hungarian paprika

- 1/2 tsp. of dried tarragon

- 1 tsp. of dried thyme

- 1/4 cup of dry vermouth

- 1 onion, chopped

- 2 garlic cloves

- 2 tbsp. of olive oil

- 1 pound of fresh porcini mushrooms, sliced

- 2 tbsp. of olive oil

- 3 cups of vegetable broth

- 1 ½ cups of white rice

Directions:

1. In a wide saucepan, put the broth and rice, add some water, and bring it to a boil.

2. Cover with a lid and turn the flame down to a low temperature and proceed to cook for the next 18 minutes or so. After cooking, let it rest for 5 to 10 minutes, and then set aside.

3. Finally, in a lightly oiled baking dish, mix the heated, fully cooked rice with the rest of your ingredients.

4. Cook at about 200° degrees for around 20 minutes in the preheated Air Fryer, regularly monitoring to even cook.

5. In small bowls, serve. Bon appétit!

13. Chinese cabbage Bake

Preparation time: 15 minutes

Cooking time: 35 minutes

Servings: 4 people

Ingredients:

- 1 cup of Monterey Jack cheese, shredded

- 1/2 tsp. of cayenne pepper

- 1 cup of cream cheese

- 1/2 cup of milk

- 4 tbsp. of flaxseed meal

- 1/2 stick butter

- 2 garlic cloves, sliced

- 1 onion, thickly sliced

- 1 jalapeno pepper, seeded and sliced

- Sea salt and freshly ground black pepper, according to taste.

- 2 bell peppers, seeded and sliced

- 1/2 pound of Chinese cabbage, roughly chopped

Directions:

1. Heat the salted water in a pan and carry it to a boil. For around 2 to 3 minutes, steam the Chinese cabbage. To end the cooking process, switch the Chinese cabbage to cold water immediately.

2. Put your Chinese cabbage in a lightly oiled casserole dish. Add in the garlic, onion, and peppers.

3. Next, over low fire, melt some butter in a skillet. Add in your flaxseed meal steadily and cook for around 2 minutes to create a paste.

4. Add in the milk gently, constantly whisking until it creates a dense mixture. Add in your cream cheese. Sprinkle some cayenne pepper, salt, and black pepper. To the casserole tray, transfer your mixture.

5. Cover with some Monterey Jack cheese and cook for about 2 minutes at around 390° F in your preheated Air Fryer. Serve it warm.

14. Brussels sprouts With Balsamic Oil

Preparation time: 5 minutes

Cooking time: 15 minutes

Servings: 4 people

Ingredients:

- 2 tbsp. of olive oil

- 2 cups of Brussels sprouts, halved

- 1 tbsp. of balsamic vinegar

- ¼ tsp. of salt

Directions:

1. For 5 minutes, preheat your air fryer.

2. In a mixing bowl, blend all of your ingredients to ensure the zucchini fries are very well coated. Put the fries in the basket of an air fryer.

3. Close it and cook it at about 350°F for around 15 minutes.

15. Aromatic Baked Potatoes with Chives

Preparation time: 15 minutes

Cooking time: 45 minutes

Servings: 2 people

Ingredients:

- 2 tbsp. of chives, chopped
- 2 garlic cloves, minced
- 1 tbsp. of sea salt
- 1/4 tsp. of smoked paprika
- 1/4 tsp. of red pepper flakes
- 2 tbsp. of olive oil
- 4 medium baking potatoes, peeled

Directions:

1. Toss the potatoes with your seasoning, olive oil, and garlic.
2. Please put them in the basket of your Air Fryer. Cook at about 400° F for around 40 minutes just until the potatoes are fork soft in your preheated Air Fryer.
3. Add in some fresh minced chives to garnish. Bon appétit!

16. Easy Vegan "chicken"

Preparation time: 10 minutes

Cooking time: 20 minutes

Servings: 4 people

Ingredients:

- 1 tsp. of celery seeds

- 1/2 tsp. of mustard powder

- 1 tsp. of cayenne pepper

- 1/4 cup of all-purpose flour

- 1/2 cup of cornmeal

- 8 ounces of soy chunks

- Sea salt and ground black pepper, according to taste.

Directions:

1. In a skillet over medium-high flame, cook the soya chunks in plenty of water. Turn off the flame and allow soaking for several minutes. Drain the remaining water, wash, and strain it out.

2. In a mixing bowl, combine the rest of the components. Roll your soy chunks over the breading paste, pressing lightly to stick.

3. In the slightly oiled Air Fryer basket, place your soy chunks.

4. Cook at about 390° for around 10 minutes in your preheated Air Fryer, rotating them over midway through the cooking process; operate in batches if required. Bon appétit!

17.Paprika Vegetable Kebab's

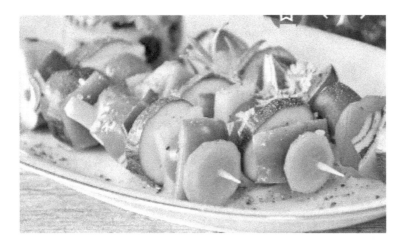

Preparation time: 10 minutes

Cooking time: 20 minutes

Servings: 4 people

Ingredients:

- 1/2 tsp. of ground black pepper

- 1 tsp. of sea salt flakes

- 1 tsp. of smoked paprika

- 1/4 cup of sesame oil

- 2 tbsp. of dry white wine

- 1 red onion, cut into wedges

- 2 cloves garlic, pressed

- 1 tsp. of whole grain mustard

- 1 fennel bulb, diced

- 1 parsnip, cut into thick slices

- 1 celery, cut into thick slices

Directions:

1. Toss all of the above ingredients together in a mixing bowl to uniformly coat. Thread the vegetables alternately onto the wooden skewers.

2. Cook for around 15 minutes at about 380° F on your Air Fryer grill plate.

3. Turn them over midway during the cooking process.

4. Taste, change the seasonings if needed and serve steaming hot.

18. Spiced Soy Curls

Preparation time: 5 minutes

Cooking time: 10 minutes

Servings: 2 people

Ingredients:

- 1 tsp. of poultry seasoning

- 2 tsp. of Cajun seasoning

- ¼ cup of fine ground cornmeal

- ¼ cup of nutritional yeast

- 4 ounces of soy curls

- 3 cups of boiling water

- Salt and ground white pepper, as needed

Directions:

1. Dip the soy curls for around a minute or so in hot water in a heat-resistant tub.

2. Drain your soy coils using a strainer and force the excess moisture out using a broad spoon.

3. Mix the cornmeal, nutritional yeast, salt, seasonings, and white pepper well in a mixing bowl.

4. Transfer your soy curls to the bowl and coat well with the blend. Let the air-fryer temperature to about 380° F. Oil the basket of your air fryers.

5. Adjust soy curls in a uniform layer in the lined air fryer basket. Cook for about 10 minutes in the air fryer, turning midway through the cycle.

6. Take out the soy curls from your air fryer and put them on a serving dish. Serve it steaming hot.

19. Cauliflower & Egg Rice Casserole

Preparation time: 5 minutes

Cooking time: 15 minutes

Servings: 4 people

Ingredients:

- 2 eggs, beaten

- 1 tablespoon of soy sauce

- Salt and black pepper according to taste.

- ½ cup of chopped onion

- 1 cup of okra, chopped

- 1 yellow bell pepper, chopped

- 2 teaspoon of olive oil

Directions:

1. Preheat your air fryer to about 380° F. Oil a baking tray with spray oil. Pulse the cauliflower till it becomes like thin rice-like capsules in your food blender.

2. Now add your cauliflower rice to a baking tray mix in the okra, bell pepper, salt, soy sauce, onion, and pepper and combine well.

3. Drizzle a little olive oil on top along with the beaten eggs. Put the tray in your air fryer and cook for about a minute. Serve it hot.

20. Hollandaise Topped Grilled Asparagus

Preparation time: 2 minutes

Cooking time: 15 minutes

Servings: 6 people

Ingredients:

- A punch of ground white pepper
- A pinch of mustard powder
- 3 pounds of asparagus spears, trimmed
- 3 egg yolks
- 2 tbsp. of olive oil
- 1 tsp. of chopped tarragon leaves
- ½ tsp. of salt
- ½ lemon juice
- ½ cup of butter, melted
- ¼ tsp. of black pepper

Directions:

1. Preheat your air fryer to about 330° F. In your air fryer, put the grill pan attachment.

2. Mix the olive oil, salt, asparagus, and pepper into a Ziploc bag. To mix all, give everything a quick shake. Load onto the grill plate and cook for about 15 minutes.

3. In the meantime, beat the lemon juice, egg yolks, and salt in a double boiler over a moderate flame until velvety.

4. Add in the melted butter, mustard powder, and some white pepper. Continue whisking till the mixture is creamy and thick. Serve with tarragon leaves as a garnish.

5. Pour the sauce over the asparagus spears and toss to blend.

21.Crispy Asparagus Dipped In Paprika-garlic Spice

Preparation time: 2 minutes

Cooking time: 15 minutes

Servings: 5 people

Ingredients:

- ¼ cup of almond flour

- ½ tsp. of garlic powder

- ½ tsp. of smoked paprika

- 10 medium asparagus, trimmed

- 2 large eggs, beaten

- 2 tbsp. of parsley, chopped

- Salt and pepper according to your taste

Directions:

1. For about 5 minutes, preheat your air fryer.

2. Mix the almond flour, garlic powder, parsley, and smoked paprika in a mixing dish. To taste, season with some salt and black pepper.

3. Soak your asparagus in the beaten eggs, and then dredge it in a combination of almond flour.

4. Put in the bowl of your air fryer. Close the lid. At about 350°F, cook for around a minute.

22. Eggplant Gratin with Mozzarella Crust

Preparation time: 10 minutes

Cooking time: 30 minutes

Servings: 2 people

Ingredients:

- 1 tablespoon of breadcrumbs

- ¼ cup of grated mozzarella cheese

- Cooking spray

- Salt and pepper according to your taste

- ¼ teaspoon of dried marjoram

- ¼ teaspoon of dried basil

- 1 teaspoon of capers

- 1 tablespoon of sliced pimiento-stuffed olives

- 1 clove garlic, minced

- ⅓ cup of chopped tomatoes

- ¼ cup of chopped onion

- ¼ cup of chopped green pepper

- ¼ cup of chopped red pepper

Directions:

1. Put the green pepper, eggplant, onion, red pepper, olives, tomatoes, basil marjoram, garlic, salt, capers, and pepper in a container and preheat your air fryer to about 300° F.

2. Lightly oil a baking tray with a spray of cooking olive oil.

3. Fill your baking with the eggplant combination and line it with the vessel.

4. Place some mozzarella cheese on top of it and top with some breadcrumbs. Put the dish in the frying pan and cook for a few minutes.

23. Asian-style Cauliflower

Preparation time: 10 minutes

Cooking time: 25 minutes

Servings: 4 people

Ingredients:

- 2 tbsp. of sesame seeds

- 1/4 cup of lime juice

- 1 tbsp. of fresh parsley, finely chopped

- 1 tbsp. of ginger, freshly grated

- 2 cloves of garlic, peeled and pressed

- 1 tbsp. of sake

- 1 tbsp. of tamari sauce

- 1 tbsp. of sesame oil

- 1 onion, peeled and finely chopped

- 2 cups of cauliflower, grated

Directions:

1. In a mixing bowl, mix your onion, cauliflower, tamari sauce, sesame oil, garlic, sake, and ginger; whisk until all is well integrated.

2. Air-fry it for around a minute at about 400° F.

3. Pause your Air Fryer. Add in some parsley and lemon juice.

4. Cook for an extra 10 minutes at about 300° degrees F in the air fryer.

5. In the meantime, in a non-stick pan, toast your sesame seeds; swirl them continuously over medium-low heat. Serve hot on top of the cauliflower with a pinch of salt and pepper.

24. Two-cheese Vegetable Frittata

Preparation time: 15 minutes

Cooking time: 35 minutes

Servings: 2 people

Ingredients:

- ⅓ cup of crumbled Feta cheese

- ⅓ cup of grated Cheddar cheese

- Salt and pepper according to taste

- ⅓ cup of milk

- 4 eggs, cracked into a bowl

- 2 teaspoon of olive oil

- ¼ lb. of asparagus, trimmed and sliced thinly

- ¼ cup of chopped chives

- 1 small red onion, sliced

- 1 large zucchini, sliced with a 1-inch thickness

- ⅓ cup of sliced mushrooms

Directions:

1. Preheat your air fryer to about 380° F. Set aside your baking dish lined with some parchment paper. Put salt, milk, and pepper into the egg bowl; whisk evenly.

2. Put a skillet on the stovetop over a moderate flame, and heat your olive oil. Add in the zucchini, asparagus, baby spinach, onion, and mushrooms; stir-fry for around 5 minutes. Transfer the vegetables into your baking tray, and finish with the beaten egg.

3. Put the tray into your air fryer and finish with cheddar and feta cheese.

4. For about 15 minutes, cook. Take out your baking tray and add in some fresh chives to garnish.

25. Rice & Beans Stuffed Bell Peppers

Preparation time: 10 minutes

Cooking time: 15 minutes

Servings: 5 people

Ingredients:

- 1 tbsp. of Parmesan cheese, grated

- ½ cup of mozzarella cheese, shredded

- 5 large bell peppers, tops removed and seeded

- 1½ tsp. of Italian seasoning

- 1 cup of cooked rice

- 1 (15-ounces) can of red kidney beans, rinsed and drained

- 1 (15-ounces) can of diced tomatoes with juice

- ½ small bell pepper, seeded and chopped

Directions:

1. Combine the tomatoes with juice, bell pepper, rice, beans, and Italian seasoning in a mixing dish. Using the rice mixture, fill each bell pepper uniformly.

2. Preheat the air fryer to 300° F. Oil the basket of your air fryer with some spray oil. Put the bell peppers in a uniform layer in your air fryer basket.

3. Cook for around 12 minutes in the air fryer. In the meantime, combine the Parmesan and mozzarella cheese in a mixing dish.

4. Remove the peppers from the air fryer basket and top each with some cheese mix. Cook for another 3 -4 minutes in the air fryer

5. Take the bell peppers from the air fryer and put them on a serving dish. Enable to cool slowly before serving. Serve it hot.

26. Parsley-loaded Mushrooms

Preparation time: 5 minutes

Cooking time: 15 minutes

Servings: 2 people

Ingredients:

- 2 tablespoon of parsley, finely chopped

- 2 teaspoon of olive oil

- 1 garlic clove, crushed

- 2 slices white bread

- salt and black pepper according to your taste

Directions:

1. Preheat the air fryer to about 360° F. Crush your bread into crumbs in a food blender. Add the parsley, garlic, and pepper; blend with the olive oil and mix.

2. Remove the stalks from the mushrooms and stuff the caps with breadcrumbs. In your air fryer basket, position the mushroom heads. Cook for a few minutes, just until golden brown and crispy.

27. Cheesy Vegetable Quesadilla

Preparation time: 2 minutes

Cooking time: 15 minutes

Servings: 1 people

Ingredients:

- 1 teaspoon of olive oil

- 1 tablespoon of cilantro, chopped

- ½ green onion, sliced

- ¼ zucchini, sliced

- ¼ yellow bell pepper, sliced

- ¼ cup of shredded gouda cheese

Directions:

1. Preheat your air fryer to about 390° F. Oil a basket of air fryers with some cooking oil.

2. Put a flour tortilla in your air fryer basket and cover it with some bell pepper, Gouda cheese, cilantro, zucchini, and green onion. Take the other tortilla to cover and spray with some olive oil.

3. Cook until slightly golden brown, for around 10 minutes. Cut into 4 slices for serving when ready. Enjoy!

28. Creamy 'n Cheese Broccoli Bake

Preparation time: 10 minutes

Cooking time: 30 minutes

Servings: 2 people

Ingredients:

- 1/4 cup of water

- 1-1/2 teaspoons of butter, or to taste

- 1/2 cup of cubed sharp Cheddar cheese

- 1/2 (14 ounces) can evaporate milk, divided

- 1/2 large onion, coarsely diced

- 1 tbsp. of dry bread crumbs, or to taste

- salt according to taste

- 2 tbsp. of all-purpose flour

- 1-pound of fresh broccoli, coarsely diced

Directions:

1. Lightly oil the air-fryer baking pan with cooking oil. Add half of the milk and flour into a pan and simmer at about 360° F for around 5 minutes.

2. Mix well midway through the cooking period. Remove the broccoli and the extra milk. Cook for the next 5 minutes after fully blending.

3. Mix in the cheese until it is fully melted. Mix the butter and bread crumbs well in a shallow tub. Sprinkle the broccoli on top.

4. At about 360° F, cook for around 20 minutes until the tops are finely golden brown. Enjoy and serve warm.

29. Sweet & Spicy Parsnips

Preparation time: 12 minutes

Cooking time: 44 minutes

Servings: 6 people

Ingredients:

- ¼ tsp. of red pepper flakes, crushed

- 1 tbsp. of dried parsley flakes, crushed

- 2 tbsp. of honey

- 1 tbsp. of n butter, melted

- 2 pounds of a parsnip, peeled and cut into 1-inch chunks

- Salt and ground black pepper, according to your taste.

Directions:

1. Let the air-fryer temperature to about 355° F. Oil the basket of your air fryers. Combine the butter and parsnips in a big dish.

2. Transfer the parsnip pieces into the lined air fryer basket arranges them in a uniform layer. Cook for a few minutes in the fryer.

3. In the meantime, combine the leftover ingredients in a large mixing bowl.

4. Move the parsnips into the honey mixture bowl after around 40 minutes and toss them to coat properly.

5. Again, in a uniform layer, organize the parsnip chunks into your air fryer basket.

6. Air-fry for another 3-4 minutes. Take the parsnip pieces from the air fryer and pass them onto the serving dish. Serve it warm.

30. Zucchini with Mediterranean Dill Sauce

Preparation time: 20 minutes

Cooking time: 60 minutes

Servings: 4 people

Ingredients:

- 1/2 tsp. of freshly cracked black peppercorns

- 2 sprigs thyme, leaves only, crushed

- 1 sprig rosemary, leaves only, crushed

- 1 tsp. of sea salt flakes

- 2 tbsp. of melted butter

- 1 pound of zucchini, peeled and cubed

For your Mediterranean Dipping:

- 1 tbsp. of olive oil

- 1 tbsp. of fresh dill, chopped

- 1/3 cup of yogurt

- 1/2 cup of mascarpone cheese

Directions:

1. To start, preheat your Air Fryer to 350° F. Now, add ice cold water to the container with your potato cubes and let them sit in the bath for about 35 minutes.

2. Dry your potato cubes with a hand towel after that. Whisk together the sea salt flakes, melted butter, thyme, rosemary, and freshly crushed peppercorns in a mixing container. This butter/spice mixture can be rubbed onto the potato cubes.

3. In the cooking basket of your air fryer, air-fry your potato cubes for around 18 to 20 minutes or until cooked completely; ensure you shake the potatoes at least once during cooking to cook them uniformly.

4. In the meantime, by mixing the rest of the ingredients, create the Mediterranean dipping sauce. To dip and eat, serve warm potatoes with Mediterranean sauce!

31. Zesty Broccoli

Preparation time: 10 minutes

Cooking time: 15 minutes

Servings: 4 people

Ingredients:

- 1 tbsp. of butter

- 1 large crown broccoli, chopped into bite-sized pieces

- 1 tbsp. of white sesame seeds

- 2 tbsp. of vegetable stock

- ½ tsp. of red pepper flakes, crushed

- 3 garlic cloves, minced

- ½ tsp. of fresh lemon zest, grated finely

- 1 tbsp. of pure lemon juice

Directions:

1. Preheat the Air fryer to about 355° F and oil an Air fryer pan with cooking spray. In the Air fryer plate, combine the vegetable stock, butter, and lemon juice.

2. Move the mixture and cook for about 2 minutes into your Air Fryer. Cook for a minute after incorporating the broccoli and garlic.

3. Cook for a minute with lemon zest, sesame seeds, and red pepper flakes. Remove the dish from the oven and eat immediately.

32. Chewy Glazed Parsnips

Preparation time: 15 minutes

Cooking time: 44 minutes

Servings: 6 people

Ingredients:

- ¼ tsp. of red pepper flakes, crushed

- 1 tbsp. of dried parsley flakes, crushed

- 2 tbsp. of maple syrup

- 1 tbsp. of butter, melted

- 2 pounds of parsnips, skinned and chopped into 1-inch chunks

Directions:

1. Preheat the Air fryer to about 355° F and oil your air fryer basket. In a wide mixing bowl, combine the butter and parsnips and toss well to cover. Cook for around 40 minutes with the parsnips in the Air fryer basket.

2. In the meantime, combine in a wide bowl the rest of your ingredients. Move this mix to your basket of the air fryer and cook for another 4 minutes or so. Remove the dish from the oven and eat promptly.

33. Hoisin-glazed Bok Choy

Preparation time: 5 minutes

Cooking time: 10 minutes

Servings: 4 people

Ingredients:

- 1 tbsp. of all-purpose flour

- 2 tbsp. of sesame oil

- 2 tbsp. of hoisin sauce

- 1/2 tsp. of sage

- 1 tsp. of onion powder

- 2 garlic cloves, minced

- 1 pound of baby Bok choy, roots removed, leaves separated

Directions:

1. In a lightly oiled Air Fryer basket, put the onion powder, garlic, Bok Choy, and sage. Cook for around 3 minutes at about 350° F in a preheated Air Fryer.

2. Whisk together the sesame oil, hoisin sauce, and flour in a deep mixing dish. Drizzle over the Bok choy with the gravy. Cook for an extra minute. Bon appétit!

34. Green Beans with Okra

Preparation time: 10 minutes

Cooking time: 20 minutes

Servings: 2 people

Ingredients:

- 3 tbsp. of balsamic vinegar

- ¼ cup of nutritional yeast

- ½ (10-ounces) of bag chilled cut green beans

- ½ (10-ounces) of bag chilled cut okra

- Salt and black pepper, according to your taste.

Directions:

1. Preheat your Air fryer to about 400° F and oil the air fryer basket.

2. In a wide mixing bowl, toss together the salt, green beans, okra, vinegar, nutritional yeast, and black pepper.

3. Cook for around 20 minutes with the okra mixture in your Air fryer basket. Dish out into a serving plate and eat warm.

35. Celeriac with some Greek Yogurt Dip

Preparation time: 12 minutes

Cooking time: 25 minutes

Servings: 2 people

Ingredients:

- 1/2 tsp. of sea salt

- 1/2 tsp. of ground black pepper, to taste

- 1 tbsp. of sesame oil

- 1 red onion, chopped into 1 1/2-inch piece

- 1/2 pound of celeriac, chopped into 1 1/2-inch piece

Spiced Yogurt:

- 1/2 tsp. of chili powder

- 1/2 tsp. of mustard seeds

- 2 tbsp. of mayonnaise

- 1/4 cup of Greek yogurt

Directions:

1. In the slightly oiled cooking basket, put the veggies in one uniform layer. Pour sesame oil over the veggies.

2. Season with a pinch of black pepper and a pinch of salt. Cook for around 20 minutes at about 300° F, tossing the basket midway through your cooking cycle.

3. In the meantime, whisk all the leftover ingredients into the sauce. Spoon the sauce over the veggies that have been cooked. Bon appétit!

36. Wine & Garlic Flavored Vegetables

Preparation time: 7-10 minutes

Cooking time: 15 minutes

Servings: 4 people

Ingredients:

- 4 cloves of garlic, minced

- 3 tbsp. of red wine vinegar

- 1/3 cup of olive oil

- 1 red onion, diced

- 1 package frozen diced vegetables

- 1 cup of baby Portobello mushrooms, diced

- 1 tsp. of Dijon mustard

- 1 ½ tbsp. of honey

- Salt and pepper according to your taste

- ¼ cup of chopped fresh basil

Directions:

1. Preheat the air fryer to about 330° F. In the air fryer, put the grill pan attachment.

2. Combine the veggies and season with pepper, salt, and garlic in a Ziploc container. To mix all, give everything a strong shake. Dump and cook for around 15 minutes on the grill pan.

3. Additionally, add the remainder of the ingredients into a mixing bowl and season with some more salt and pepper. Drizzle the sauce over your grilled vegetables.

37. Spicy Braised Vegetables

Preparation time: 10 minutes

Cooking time: 25 minutes

Servings: 4 people

Ingredients:

- 1/2 cup of tomato puree

- 1/4 tsp. of ground black pepper

- 1/2 tsp. of fine sea salt

- 1 tbsp. of garlic powder

- 1/2 tsp. of fennel seeds

- 1/4 tsp. of mustard powder

- 1/2 tsp. of porcini powder

- 1/4 cup of olive oil

- 1 celery stalk, chopped into matchsticks

- 2 bell peppers, deveined and thinly diced

- 1 Serrano pepper, deveined and thinly diced

- 1 large-sized zucchini, diced

Directions:

1. In your Air Fryer cooking basket, put your peppers, zucchini, sweet potatoes, and carrot.

2. Drizzle with some olive oil and toss to cover completely; cook for around 15 minutes in a preheated Air Fryer at about 350°F.

3. Make the sauce as the vegetables are frying by quickly whisking the remaining ingredients (except the tomato ketchup). Slightly oil up a baking dish that fits your fryer.

4. Add the cooked vegetables to the baking dish, along with the sauce, and toss well to cover.

5. Turn the Air Fryer to about 390° F and cook for 2-4 more minutes with the vegetables. Bon appétit!

CHAPTER 3: Air Fryer Snack Side Dishes and Appetizer Recipes

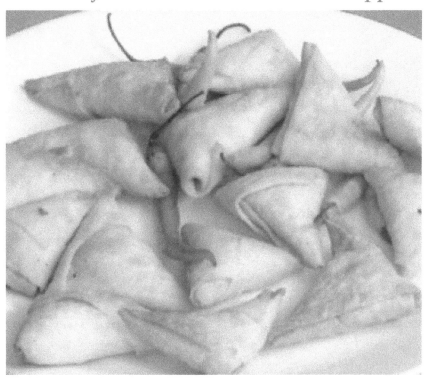

1. Crispy 'n Tasty Spring Rolls

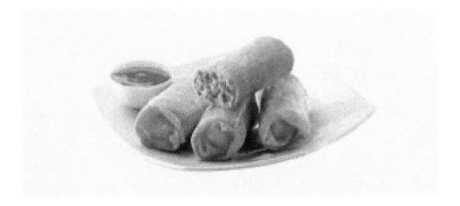

Preparation time: 5 minutes

Cooking time: 15 minutes

Servings: 4 people

Ingredients:

- 8 spring roll wrappers

- 1 tsp. of nutritional yeast

- 1 tsp. of corn starch + 2 tablespoon water

- 1 tsp. of coconut sugar

- 1 tbsp. of soy sauce

- 1 medium carrot, shredded

- 1 cup of shiitake mushroom, sliced thinly

- 1 celery stalk, chopped

- ½ tsp. of ginger, finely chopped

Directions:

1. Mix your carrots, celery stalk, soy sauce, coconut sugar, ginger, and nutritional yeast with each other in a mixing dish.

2. Have a tbsp. of your vegetable mix and put it in the middle of your spring roll wrappers.

3. Roll up and secure the sides of your wraps with some cornstarch.

4. Cook for about 15 minutes or till your spring roll wraps is crisp in a preheated air fryer at 200F.

2. Spinach & Feta Crescent Triangles

Preparation time: 10 minutes

Cooking time: 20 minutes

Servings: 4 people

Ingredients:

- ¼ teaspoon of salt

- 1 teaspoon of chopped oregano

- ¼ teaspoon of garlic powder

- 1 cup of crumbled feta cheese

- 1 cup of steamed spinach

Directions:

1. Preheat your air fryer to about 350 F, and then roll up the dough over a level surface that is gently floured.

2. In a medium-sized bowl, mix the spinach, feta, salt, oregano, and ground garlic cloves. Split your dough into four equal chunks.

3. Split the mix of feta/spinach among the four chunks of dough. Fold and seal your dough using a fork.

4. Please put it on a baking tray covered with parchment paper, and then put it in your air fryer.

5. Cook until nicely golden, for around 1 minute.

3. Healthy Avocado Fries

Preparation time: 5 minutes

Cooking time: 20 minutes

Servings: 2 people

Ingredients:

- ¼ cup of aquafaba

- 1 avocado, cubed

- Salt as required

Directions:

1. Mix the aquafaba, crumbs, and salt in a mixing bowl.

2. Preheat your air fryer to about 390°F and cover the avocado pieces uniformly in the crumbs blend.

3. Put the ready pieces in the cooking bucket of your air fryer and cook for several minutes.

4. Twice-fried Cauliflower Tater Tots

Preparation time: 5 minutes

Cooking time: 16 minutes

Servings: 12 people

Ingredients:

- 3 tbsp. Of oats flaxseed meal + 3 tbsp. of water)

- 1-pound of cauliflower, steamed and chopped

- 1 tsp. of parsley, chopped

- 1 tsp. of oregano, chopped

- 1 tsp. of garlic, minced

- 1 tsp. of chives, chopped

- 1 onion, chopped

- 1 flax egg (1 tablespoon 3 tablespoon desiccated coconuts)

- ½ cup of nutritional yeast

- salt and pepper according to taste

- ½ cup of bread crumbs

Directions:

1. Preheat your air fryer to about 390 degrees F.

2. To extract extra moisture, place the steamed cauliflower onto a ring and a paper towel.

3. Put and mix the remainder of your ingredients, excluding your bread crumbs, in a small mixing container.

4. Use your palms, blend it until well mixed and shapes into a small ball.

5. Roll your tater tots over your bread crumbs and put them in the bucket of your air fryer.

6. For a minute, bake. Raise the cooking level to about 400 F and cook for the next 10 minutes.

5. Cheesy Mushroom & Cauliflower Balls

Preparation time: 10 minutes

Cooking time: 50 minutes

Servings: 4 people

Ingredients:

- Salt and pepper according to taste

- 2 sprigs chopped fresh thyme

- ¼ cup of coconut oil

- 1 cup of Grana Padano cheese

- 1 cup of breadcrumbs

- 2 tablespoon of vegetable stock

- 3 cups of cauliflower, chopped

- 3 cloves garlic, minced

- 1 small red onion, chopped

- 3 tablespoon of olive oil

Directions:

1. Over moderate flame, put a pan. Add some balsamic vinegar. When the oil is heated, stir-fry your onion and garlic till they become transparent.

2. Add in the mushrooms and cauliflower and stir-fry for about 5 minutes. Add in your stock, add thyme and cook till your cauliflower has consumed the stock. Add pepper, Grana Padano cheese, and salt.

3. Let the mix cool down and form bite-size spheres of your paste. To harden, put it in the fridge for about 30 minutes.

4. Preheat your air fryer to about 350°F.

5. Add your coconut oil and breadcrumbs into a small bowl and blend properly.

6. Take out your mushroom balls from the fridge, swirl the breadcrumb paste once more, and drop the balls into your breadcrumb paste.

7. Avoid overcrowding, put your balls into your air fryer's container and cook for about 15 minutes, flipping after every 5 minutes to ensure even cooking.

8. Serve with some tomato sauce and brown sugar.

6. Italian Seasoned Easy Pasta Chips

Preparation time: 5 minutes

Cooking time: 10 minutes

Servings: 2 people

Ingredients:

- 2 cups of whole wheat bowtie pasta

- 1 tbsp. of olive oil

- 1 tbsp. of nutritional yeast

- 1 ½ tsp. of Italian seasoning blend

- ½ tsp. of salt

Directions:

1. Put the accessory for the baking tray into your air fryer.

2. Mix all the ingredients in a medium-sized bowl, offer it a gentle stir.

3. Add the mixture to your air fryer basket.

4. Close your air fryer and cook at around 400°degrees F for about 10 minutes.

7. Thai Sweet Potato Balls

Preparation time: 10 minutes

Cooking time: 50 minutes

Servings: 4 people

Ingredients:

- 1 cup of coconut flakes

- 1 tsp. of baking powder

- 1/2 cup of almond meal

- 1/4 tsp. of ground cloves

- 1/2 tsp. of ground cinnamon

- 2 tsp. of orange zest

- 1 tbsp. of orange juice

- 1 cup of brown sugar

- 1 pound of sweet potatoes

Directions:

1. Bake your sweet potatoes for around 25 to 30 minutes at about 380° F till they become soft; peel and mash them in a medium-sized bowl.

2. Add orange zest, orange juice, brown sugar, ground cinnamon, almond meal, cloves, and baking powder. Now blend completely.

3. Roll the balls around in some coconut flakes.

4. Bake for around 15 minutes or until fully fried and crunchy in the preheated Air Fryer at about 360° F.

5. For the rest of the ingredients, redo the same procedure. Bon appétit!

8. Barbecue Roasted Almonds

Preparation time: 5 minutes

Cooking time: 20 minutes

Servings: 6 people

Ingredients:

- 1 tbsp. of olive oil

- 1/4 tsp. of smoked paprika

- 1/2 tsp. of cumin powder

- 1/4 tsp. of mustard powder

- 1/4 tsp. of garlic powder

- Sea salt and ground black pepper, according to taste

- 1 ½ cups of raw almonds

Directions:

1. In a mixing pot, mix all your ingredients.

2. Line the container of your Air Fryer with some baking parchment paper. Arrange the covered almonds out in the basket of your air fryer in a uniform layer.

3. Roast for around 8 to 9 minutes at about 340°F, tossing the bucket once or twice. If required, work in groups.

4. Enjoy!

9. Croissant Rolls

Preparation time: 2 minutes

Cooking time: 6 minutes

Servings: 8 people

Ingredients:

- 4 tbsp. of butter, melted

- 1 (8-ounces) can croissant rolls

Directions:

1. Adjust the air-fryer temperature to about 320°F. Oil the basket of your air fryers.

2. Into your air fryer basket, place your prepared croissant rolls.

3. Airs fry them for around 4 minutes or so.

4. Flip to the opposite side and cook for another 2-3 minutes.

5. Take out from your air fryer and move to a tray.

6. Glaze with some melted butter and eat warm.

10.Curry' n Coriander Spiced Bread Rolls

Preparation time: 5 minutes

Cooking time: 15 minutes

Servings: 5 people

Ingredients:

- salt and pepper according to taste

- 5 large potatoes, boiled

- 2 sprigs, curry leaves

- 2 small onions, chopped

- 2 green chilies, seeded and chopped

- 1 tbsp. of olive oil

- 1 bunch of coriander, chopped

- ½ tsp. of turmeric

- 8 slices of vegan wheat bread, brown sides discarded

- ½ tsp. of mustard seeds

Directions:

1. Mash your potatoes in a bowl and sprinkle some black pepper and salt according to taste. Now set aside.

2. In a pan, warm up the olive oil over medium-low heat and add some mustard seeds. Mix until the seeds start to sputter.

3. Now add in the onions and cook till they become transparent. Mix in the curry leaves and turmeric powder.

4. Keep on cooking till it becomes fragrant for a couple of minutes. Take it off the flame and add the mixture to the potatoes.

5. Mix in the green chilies and some coriander. This is meant to be the filling.

6. Wet your bread and drain excess moisture. In the center of the loaf, put a tbsp. of the potato filling and gently roll the bread so that the potato filling is fully enclosed within the bread.

7. Brush with some oil and put them inside your air fryer basket.

8. Cook for around 15 minutes in a preheated air fryer at about 400°F.

9. Ensure that the air fryer basket is shaken softly midway through the cooking period for an even cooking cycle.

11. Scrumptiously Healthy Chips

Preparation time: 5 minutes

Cooking time: 10 minutes

Servings: 2 people

Ingredients:

- 2 tbsp. of olive oil

- 2 tbsp. of almond flour

- 1 tsp. of garlic powder

- 1 bunch kale

- Salt and pepper according to taste

Directions:

1. For around 5 minutes, preheat your air fryer.

2. In a mixing bowl, add all your ingredients, add the kale leaves at the end and toss to completely cover them.

3. Put in the basket of your fryer and cook until crispy for around 10 minutes.

12. Kid-friendly Vegetable Fritters

Preparation time: 5 minutes

Cooking time: 20 minutes

Servings: 4 people

Ingredients:

- 2 tbsp. of olive oil

- 1/2 cup of cornmeal

- 1/2 cup of all-purpose flour

- 1/2 tsp. of ground cumin

- 1 tsp. of turmeric powder

- 2 garlic cloves, pressed

- 1 carrot, grated

- 1 sweet pepper, seeded and chopped

- 1 yellow onion, finely chopped

- 1 tbsp. of ground flaxseeds

- Salt and ground black pepper, according to taste

- 1 pound of broccoli florets

Directions:

1. In salted boiling water, blanch your broccoli until al dente, for around 3 to 5 minutes. Drain the excess water and move to a mixing bowl; add in the rest of your ingredients to mash the broccoli florets.

2. Shape the paste into patties and position them in the slightly oiled Air Fryer basket.

3. Cook for around 6 minutes at about 400° F, flipping them over midway through the cooking process; if needed, operate in batches.

4. Serve hot with some Vegenaise of your choice. Enjoy it!

13. Avocado Fries

Preparation time: 10 minutes

Cooking time: 50 minutes

Servings: 4 people

Ingredients:

- 2 avocados, cut into wedges

- 1/2 cup of parmesan cheese, grated

- 2 eggs

- Sea salt and ground black pepper, according to taste.

- 1/2 cup of almond meal

- 1/2 head garlic (6-7 cloves)

Sauce:

- 1 tsp. of mustard

- 1 tsp. of lemon juice

- 1/2 cup of mayonnaise

Directions:

1. On a piece of aluminum foil, put your garlic cloves and spray some cooking spray on it. Wrap your garlic cloves in the foil.

2. Cook for around 1-2 minutes at about 400°F in your preheated Air Fryer. Inspect the garlic, open the foil's top end, and keep cooking for an additional 10-12 minutes.

3. Once done, let them cool for around 10 to 15 minutes; take out the cloves by pressing them out of their skin; mash your garlic and put them aside.

4. Mix the salt, almond meal, and black pepper in a small dish.

5. Beat the eggs until foamy in a separate bowl.

6. Put some parmesan cheese in the final shallow dish.

7. In your almond meal blend, dip the avocado wedges, dusting off any excess.

8. In the beaten egg, dunk your wedges; eventually, dip in some parmesan cheese.

9. Spray your avocado wedges on both sides with some cooking oil spray.

10. Cook for around 8 minutes in the preheated Air Fryer at about 395° F, flipping them over midway thru the cooking process.

11. In the meantime, mix the ingredients of your sauce with your cooked crushed garlic.

12. Split the avocado wedges between plates and cover with the sauce before serving. Enjoy!

14. Crispy Wings with Lemony Old Bay Spice

Preparation time: 10 minutes

Cooking time: 25 minutes

Servings: 4 people

Ingredients:

- Salt and pepper according to taste

- 3 pounds of vegan chicken wings

- 1 tsp. of lemon juice, freshly squeezed

- 1 tbsp. of old bay spices

- ¾ cup of almond flour

- ½ cup of butter

Directions:

1. For about 5 minutes, preheat your air fryer. Mix all your ingredients in a mixing dish, excluding the butter. Put in the bowl of an air fryer.

2. Preheat the oven to about 350°F and bake for around 25 minutes. Rock the fryer container midway thru the cooking process, also for cooking.

3. Drizzle with some melted butter when it's done frying. Enjoy!

15. Cold Salad with Veggies and Pasta

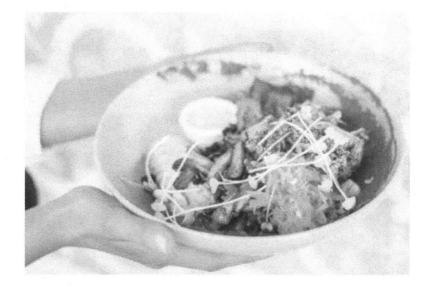

Preparation time: 30 minutes

Cooking time: 1 hour 35 minutes

Servings: 12 people

Ingredients:

- ½ cup of fat-free Italian dressing

- 2 tablespoons of olive oil, divided

- ½ cup of Parmesan cheese, grated

- 8 cups of cooked pasta

- 4 medium tomatoes, cut in eighths

- 3 small eggplants, sliced into ½-inch thick rounds

- 3 medium zucchinis, sliced into ½-inch thick rounds

- Salt, according to your taste.

Directions:

1. Preheat your Air fryer to about 355° F and oil the inside of your air fryer basket. In a dish, mix 1 tablespoon of olive oil and zucchini and swirl to cover properly.

2. Cook for around 25 minutes your zucchini pieces in your Air fryer basket. In another dish, mix your eggplants with a tablespoon of olive oil and toss to coat properly.

3. Cook for around 40 minutes your eggplant slices in your Air fryer basket. Re-set the Air Fryer temperature to about 320° F and put the tomatoes next in the ready basket.

4. Cook and mix all your air-fried vegetables for around 30 minutes. To serve, mix in the rest of the ingredients and chill for at least 2 hours, covered.

16. Zucchini and Minty Eggplant Bites

Preparation time: 15 minutes

Cooking time: 35 minutes

Servings: 8 people

Ingredients:

- 3 tbsp. of olive oil

- 1 pound of zucchini, peeled and cubed

- 1 pound of eggplant, peeled and cubed

- 2 tbsp. of melted butter

- 1 ½ tsp. of red pepper chili flakes

- 2 tsp. of fresh mint leaves, minced

Directions:

1. In a large mixing container, add all of the ingredients mentioned above.

2. Roast the zucchini bites and eggplant in your Air Fryer for around 30 minutes at about 300° F, flipping once or twice during the cooking cycle. Serve with some dipping sauce that's homemade.

17. Stuffed Potatoes

Preparation time: 15 minutes

Cooking time: 31 minutes

Servings: 4 people

Ingredients:

- 3 tbsp. of canola oil

- ½ cup of Parmesan cheese, grated

- 2 tbsp. of chives, chopped

- ½ of brown onion, chopped

- 1 tbsp. of butter

- 4 potatoes, peeled

Directions:

1. Preheat the Air fryer to about 390° F and oil the air fryer basket. Coat the canola oil on the potatoes and place them in your Air Fryer Basket.

2. Cook for around 20 minutes before serving on a platter. Halve each potato and scrape out the middle from each half of it.

3. In a frying pan, melt some butter over medium heat and add the onions. Sauté in a bowl for around 5 minutes and dish out.

4. Combine the onions with the middle of the potato, chives and half of the cheese. Stir well and uniformly cram the onion potato mixture into the potato halves.

5. Top and layer the potato halves in your Air Fryer basket with the leftover cheese. Cook for around 6 minutes before serving hot.

18.Paneer Cutlet

Preparation time: 5 minutes

Cooking time: 15 minutes

Servings: 1 people

Ingredients:

- ½ teaspoon of salt

- ½ teaspoon of oregano

- 1 small onion, finely chopped

- ½ teaspoon of garlic powder

- 1 teaspoon of butter

- ½ teaspoon of chai masala

- 1 cup of grated cheese

Directions:

1. Preheat the air fryer to about 350° F and lightly oil a baking dish. In a mixing bowl, add all ingredients and stir well. Split the mixture into cutlets and put them in an oiled baking dish.

2. Put the baking dish in your air fryer and cook your cutlets until crispy, around a minute or so.

19.Spicy Roasted Cashew Nuts

Preparation time: 10 Minutes

Cooking time: 20 Minutes

Servings: 4

Ingredients:

- 1/2 tsp. of ancho chili powder

- 1/2 tsp. of smoked paprika

- Salt and ground black pepper, according to taste

- 1 tsp. of olive oil

- 1 cup of whole cashews

Directions:

1. In a mixing big bowl, toss all your ingredients.

2. Line parchment paper to cover the Air Fryer container. Space out the spiced cashews in your basket in a uniform layer.

3. Roast for about 6 to 8 minutes at 300 degrees F, tossing the basket once or twice during the cooking process. Work in batches if needed. Enjoy!

CHAPTER 4: Deserts

1. Almond-apple Treat

Preparation time: 5 minutes

Cooking time: 15 minutes

Servings: 4 people

Ingredients:

- 2 tablespoon of sugar

- ¾ oz. of raisins

- 1 ½ oz. of almonds

Directions:

1. Preheat your air fryer to around 360° F.

2. Mix the almonds, sugar, and raisins in a dish. Blend using a hand mixer.

3. Load the apples with a combination of the almond mixture. Please put them in the air fryer basket and cook for a few minutes. Enjoy!

2. Pepper-pineapple With Butter-sugar Glaze

Preparation time: 5 minutes

Cooking time: 10 minutes

Servings: 2 people

Ingredients:

- Salt according to taste.

- 2 tsp. of melted butter

- 1 tsp. of brown sugar

- 1 red bell pepper, seeded and julienned

- 1 medium-sized pineapple, peeled and sliced

Directions:

1. To about 390°F, preheat your air fryer. In your air fryer, put the grill pan attachment.

2. In a Ziploc bag, combine all ingredients and shake well.

3. Dump and cook on the grill pan for around 10 minutes to ensure you turn the pineapples over every 5 minutes during cooking.

3. True Churros with Yummy Hot Chocolate

Preparation time: 10 minutes

Cooking time: 25 minutes

Servings: 3 people

Ingredients:

- 1 tsp. of ground cinnamon

- 1/3 cup of sugar

- 1 tbsp. of cornstarch

- 1 cup of milk

- 2 ounces of dark chocolate

- 1 cup of all-purpose flour

- 1 tbsp. of canola oil

- 1 tsp. of lemon zest

- 1/4 tsp. of sea salt

- 2 tbsp. of granulated sugar

- 1/2 cup of water

Directions:

1. To create the churro dough, boil the water in a pan over a medium-high flame; then, add the salt, sugar, and lemon zest and fry, stirring continuously, until fully dissolved.

2. Take the pan off the heat and add in some canola oil. Stir the flour in steadily, constantly stirring until the solution turns to a ball.

3. With a broad star tip, pipe the paste into a piping bag. In the oiled Air Fryer basket, squeeze 4-inch slices of dough. Cook for around 6 minutes at a temperature of 300° F.

4. Make the hot cocoa for dipping in the meantime. In a shallow saucepan, melt some chocolate and 1/2 cup of milk over low flame.

5. In the leftover 1/2 cup of milk, mix the cornstarch and blend it into the hot chocolate mixture. Cook for around 5 minutes on low flame.

6. Mix the sugar and cinnamon; roll your churros in this combination. Serve with a side of hot cocoa. Enjoy!

Conclusion

These times, air frying is one of the most common cooking techniques and air fryers have become one of the chef's most impressive devices. In no time, air fryers can help you prepare nutritious and tasty meals! To prepare unique dishes for you and your family members, you do not need to be a master in the kitchen.

Everything you have to do is buy an air fryer and this wonderful cookbook for air fryers! Soon, you can make the greatest dishes ever and inspire those around you.

Cooked meals at home with you! Believe us! Get your hands on an air fryer and this handy set of recipes for air fryers and begin your new cooking experience. Have fun!

CPSIA information can be obtained
at www.ICGtesting.com
Printed in the USA
BVHW061701200521
607638BV00018B/634